HPNA PALLIATIVE NURSING MANUALS

Physical Aspects
of Care

HPNA PALLIATIVE NURSING MANUALS

Series edited by: Betty R. Ferrell, RN, PhD, MA, FAAN, FPCN, CHPN

Volume 1: Structure and Processes of Care

Volume 2: Physical Aspects of Care: Pain and Gastrointestinal Symptoms

Volume 3: Physical Aspects of Care: Nutritional, Dermatologic, Neurologic, and Other Symptoms

Volume 4: Pediatric Palliative Care

Volume 5: Social Aspects of Care

Volume 6: Spiritual, Religious, and Existential Aspects of Care and Cultural Aspects

Volume 7: Care of the Patient at the End of Life

Volume 8: Ethical and Legal Aspects of Care

HPNA PALLIATIVE NURSING MANUALS

Physical Aspects of Care: Nutritional, Dermatologic, Neurologic, and Other Symptoms

Edited by

Judith A. Paice, PhD, RN, FAAN

Director of Cancer Pain Program
Division of Hematology-Oncology
Feinberg School of Medicine
Northwestern University
Chicago, Illinois

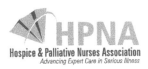

Hospice & Palliative Nurses Association
Advancing Expert Care in Serious Illness

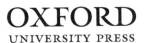

OXFORD
UNIVERSITY PRESS

OXFORD

UNIVERSITY PRESS

Oxford University Press is a department of the University of
Oxford. It furthers the University's objective of excellence in research,
scholarship, and education by publishing worldwide.

Oxford   New York
Auckland   Cape Town   Dar es Salaam   Hong Kong   Karachi
Kuala Lumpur   Madrid   Melbourne   Mexico City   Nairobi
New Delhi   Shanghai   Taipei   Toronto

With offices in
Argentina   Austria   Brazil   Chile   Czech Republic   France   Greece
Guatemala   Hungary   Italy   Japan   Poland   Portugal   Singapore
South Korea   Switzerland   Thailand   Turkey   Ukraine   Vietnam

Oxford is a registered trademark of Oxford University Press
in the UK and certain other countries.

Published in the United States of America by
Oxford University Press
198 Madison Avenue, New York, NY 10016

Library of Congress Cataloging-in-Publication Data
Physical aspects of care. Nutritional, dermatologic, neurologic, and other symptoms / edited by
Judith A. Paice.
p. ; cm.—(HPNA palliative nursing manuals ; v. 3)
Nutritional, dermatologic, neurologic, and other symptoms
"Content for this series was derived primarily from the Oxford Textbook of Palliative Nursing
(4th edition, 2015), edited by Betty R. Ferrell, Nessa Coyle, Judith A. Paice. The Textbook contains
more extensive content and references so users of this Palliative Nursing Series are encouraged
to use the Textbook as an additional resource."—Preface.
Includes bibliographical references and index.
ISBN 978–0–19–024433–0 (alk. paper)
I. Paice, Judith A., editor.   II. Oxford textbook of palliative nursing. 4th edition. 2014.
Based on (expression):   III. Title: Nutritional, dermatologic, neurologic, and other symptoms.
IV. Series: HPNA palliative nursing manuals ; v. 3.
[DNLM: 1. Hospice and Palliative Care Nursing.   2. Neurologic Manifestations.   3. Nutrition
Disorders—nursing.   4. Palliative Care—methods.   5. Skin Diseases—nursing.   6. Terminal
Care—methods. WY 152.3]
R726.8
616.02′9—dc23
2014047648

9 8 7 6 5 4 3 2
Printed in Canada

Contents

Preface

This is the third volume of a new series being published by Oxford University Press in collaboration with the Hospice and Palliative Nurses Association. The intent of this series is to provide palliative care nurses with quick reference guides to each of the key domains of palliative care.

Content for this series was derived primarily from the *Oxford Textbook of Palliative Nursing* (4th edition, 2015), which is also edited by Betty Ferrell, the editor of this series, Nessa Coyle, and Judith Paice. The Contributors identified in each volume are the authors of chapters in the *Oxford Textbook of Palliative Nursing* from which the content was selected for this volume. The Textbook contains more extensive content and references, so users of this Palliative Nursing Series are encouraged to use the Textbook as an additional resource.

We are grateful to all palliative care nurses who are contributing to the advancement of care for seriously ill patients and families. Remarkable progress has occurred over the past 30 years in this field, and nurses have been central to that progress. Our hope is that this series offers an additional tool to build the care delivery system we strive for.

Contributors

Paula R. Anderson, RN, MN, OCN
Oncology Research Initiatives
University of Texas Southwestern
    Medical Center
Moncrief Cancer Center
Fort Worth, Texas

Barbara M. Bates-Jensen, PhD, RN, FAAN
Associate Professor of Nursing
School of Nursing and David Geffen
    School of Medicine
University of California, Los Angeles
Los Angeles, California

Laura Bourdeanu, PhD
Assistant Professor of Nursing
The Sage Colleges
Troy, New York

Grace E. Dean, PhD, RN
Postdoctoral Fellow
School of Nursing
Center for Sleep and Respiratory
    Neurobiology
University of Pennsylvania
Philadelphia, Pennsylvania

Mei R. Fu, PhD, RN, ACNS-BC, FAAN
College of Nursing
New York University
New York, New York

Michelle S. Gabriel, RN, MS, ACHPN
VA Palo Alto Health Care System
Palo Alto, California

Mikel Gray, PhD
Professor of Nursing
Department of Acute and
    Specialty Care
University of Virginia
Charlottesville, Virginia

Marjorie J. Hein, MSN
Nurse Practitioner
Nursing Support, Medical Oncology
City of Hope National
    Medical Center
Duarte, California

Philip J. Larkin, BSc, MSc, PhD
Professor of Clinical Nursing
School of Nursing, Midwifery and
    Health Systems
University College Dublin
Belfield, Ireland

Ellen A. Liu, MSN
Nurse Practitioner
City of Hope National
    Medical Center
Duarte, California

Pamela A. Minarik, MS, APRN, BC, FAAN
Professor of Nursing
Professor, Office of International
    Affairs
Yale University School of Nursing
Psychiatric Consultation Liaison
    Clinical Nurse Specialist
Yale-New Haven Hospital
New Haven, Connecticut

ix

Edith O'Neil-Page, RN, MSN, AOCNS

Palliative Care Clinical Nurse
    Specialist
UCLA Ronald Reagan Medical Center
Los Angeles, California

Leslie Nield-Anderson, ARNP, PhD

Geropsychiatric Consultant
Sunhill Medical Center
Sun City Center, Florida

Jeannie V. Pasacreta, PhD, APRN, CEO

Integrated Mental Health
    Services, LLC
Newtown, Connecticut

Sirin Petch, RN

Clinical Nurse
University of California, Los Angeles
Los Angeles, California

Margaret A. Schwartz, MSN, CNRN, APN

Department of Neurology
Northwestern University
Chicago, Illinois

Susie Seaman, NP, MSN, CWOCN

Sharp Rees-Stealy Wound Clinic
San Diego, California

Terran Sims, RN, MSN, ACNP

Nurse Practitioner
Department of Urology
University of Virginia
Charlottesville, Virginia

Jennifer A. Tschanz, RN, MSN, FNP, AOCNP

Nurse Practitioner
Department of Hematology
    Oncology
Naval Medical Center
San Diego, California

Dorothy Wholihan, DNP, ANP-BC, GNP-BC, ACHPN

Clinical Assistant Professor of
    Nursing
Coordinator of Palliative Care
New York University
New York, New York

Chapter 1

Fatigue

Edith O'Neil-Page, Paula R. Anderson and Grace E. Dean

Introduction

Fatigue is a devastating, multidimensional symptom that involves the entire person, touching every facet of daily life. It can progressively interfere with a patient's physical and social activities, resulting in increased withdrawal. Fatigue is a symptom that possibly has the greatest potential to interfere with quality of life at the end of life. Fatigue has been reported to be the most common symptom that is linked to the clinical course of cancer and other chronic diseases. Estimates of its prevalence are between 60% and 90%.

Fatigue is described as a lack of energy or exhaustion that frequently interferes with normal activities and function and for which affect and/or manifestation differ with diagnosis and/or treatment. In oncology, for example, patients perceive fatigue differently depending on where in the disease trajectory fatigue occurs. It is often the recognition of symptoms that causes the patient with an undiagnosed cancer to seek medical treatment. Once diagnosed, the cancer patient experiences fatigue as a side effect of treatment. Pervasive, cancer-related fatigue presents across stages of the disease process and often continues well into recovery. The patient who has finished treatment and is in recovery discovers a "new normal" level of energy. The patient who has experienced a recurrence of cancer considers fatigue to be as much an enemy as the diagnosis itself. Finally, the patient who is in the advanced stages of cancer interprets fatigue as the end of a very long struggle, as something to be endured.

The National Comprehensive Cancer Network (NCCN) Fatigue Practice Guidelines Panel defines fatigue as "a distressing, persistent, subjective sense of physical, emotional and/or cognitive tiredness or exhaustion related to cancer or cancer treatment that is not proportional to recent activity and interferes with usual functioning."[1] The European Association for Palliative Care identified a working definition of fatigue as a subjective feeling of tiredness, weakness, or lack of energy.[2] Although other definitions have been proposed, the two key elements that are dominant in most definitions of fatigue are (1) subjective perception with physical, emotional, and cognitive features; and (2) interference with the ability to function.

Pathophysiology

Models to explain the causes of fatigue have been developed by a variety of disciplines in the basic sciences and by clinicians. The two most prominent constructs are the depletion hypothesis and the accumulation hypothesis. In the *depletion hypothesis,* essential substances integral to muscle activity are not available or have been depleted, causing fatigue. The *accumulation hypothesis* describes a mechanism whereby waste products collect and outpace the body's ability to dispose of them, resulting in fatigue.

Recent evidence suggests that pro-inflammatory cytokines may play a mechanistic role in the symptom of fatigue as a common biologic mechanism.[3,4] A constellation of physiologic and behavioral responses observed in animals, termed *sickness behavior* (hyperalgesia, sleep disturbance, reduced activity, reduction in food intake), can be elicited by bacterial infections and administration of lipopolysaccharides-pathologic components of bacteria.[3] In humans, pro-inflammatory cytokines may be released as part of the host response to infection, a tumor, tissue damage from injury, or depletion of immune cells associated with treatments.[3] These inflammatory stimuli can signal the central nervous system to generate fatigue, as well as changes in sleep, appetite, reproduction, and social behavior.

Fatigue, like pain, not only is explained by physiologic mechanisms but also must be understood as a multi-causal, multidimensional phenomenon that includes physical, psychological, social, and spiritual aspects. As such, factors influencing fatigue are beginning to be addressed.

Factors Influencing Fatigue

Characteristics that may predispose patients with advanced disease to develop fatigue have not been comprehensively studied. Oncology research has placed importance on patient characteristics in treatment-related fatigue. Box 1.1 provides a list of factors that have been associated with cancer-related fatigue as well as other terminal diseases.

Younger adult patients with cancer report more fatigue than older patients.[5] This suggests that fatigue may be influenced by the developmental level of the adult. For example, young adults may have heavy responsibilities of balancing career, marriage, and childrearing, whereas older adults may be at the end of their careers or retired with "empty nests." Additionally, the older adult often has more than one simultaneous medical condition and may attribute the fatigue to advancing age and view the fatigue as normal. These may partially explain why studies report that younger adults have fatigue more frequently. However, in a study of cancer patients aged 70 to 90 years, it was reported that fatigue was a long-lasting complication of cancer and treatment and might actually have caused as well as accelerated these elderly patients' functional decline.[6] More recent studies indicate that an increase in prevalence of cancer in elderly people, accompanied by other chronic disease and stress associated with multiple treatments, predisposes elderly people to fatigue.

Box 1.1 Factors Associated With Fatigue Development

Personal Factors

Age (developmental stage)
Marital status (home demands, isolation)
Menopausal status
Income and insurance

Psychosocial Factors

Mental and emotional state (depression, fear, anxiety, distress, conflicts)
Culture and ethnicity
Living situation

Care-Related Factors

Number and cohesiveness of caregivers
Responsiveness of health care providers

Disease-Related Factors

Stage and extent of disease
Comorbidities
Anemia
Pain
Dyspnea
Nutritional changes (weight loss, cachexia, electrolyte imbalance)
Continence
Sleep patterns and interruptions

Treatment-Related Factors

Any treatment-related effect from surgery, chemotherapy, or radiation (skin reaction, temporary altered energy level, urinary and bowel changes, pain)
Medication issues (side effects, polypharmacy, taste changes, over-the-counter medications)
Permanent physiologic changes

Depression has been linked to patients with cancer-related fatigue.[7] Depression and fatigue are two related concepts. Fatigue is part of the diagnostic criteria for depression, and depression may develop as a result of being fatigued. Although depression is less frequently reported than fatigue, feelings of depression are common in patients with cancer, with a prevalence rate in the range of 20% to 25%. One study exploring correlates of fatigue found a fused relationship between depression and fatigue. This research indicated that fatigued women scored twice as high on the depression scale as those who were not fatigued and also that depression was the strongest predictor of fatigue. Additionally, depression and fatigue may coexist with cancer without having a causal relationship because each can originate from the same pathology.

Fatigue in patients undergoing cancer treatment has been closely linked with other distressing symptoms, such as pain, dyspnea, anorexia, constipation, sleep disruption, depression, anxiety, and other mood states. Research on patients with advanced cancer has demonstrated that fatigue severity was significantly associated with similar symptoms.

Assessment

Fatigue assessment of the whole person is essential, including the mind and spirit as well as the body.[8,9] There is no agreement on one definition for fatigue—it is the patient's definition or description of fatigue that counts. This personal fatigue may include any reference to a decrease in energy, weakness, or a tired or "wiped out" feeling. What's important is that the concept of fatigue is valued, evaluated, and described to enable appropriate responses. Box 1.2 lists proposed criteria for diagnosing cancer-related fatigue.[10]

There are numerous methods of assessing and diagnosing fatigue. Many scales have been developed to measure fatigue in the adult, with varying levels

---

Box 1.2 Proposed Criteria for Diagnosing Cancer-Related Fatigue

These symptoms have been present almost every day during the same 2-week period in the past month:

Significant fatigue, diminished energy, or increased need of rest, disproportionate to any recent change in activity, as well as five or more of the following:

1. Complaints of generalized weakness or limb heaviness
2. Diminished concentration or attention
3. Decreased motivation or interest in engaging in usual activities
4. Insomnia or hypersomnia
5. Sleep that is unrefreshing or nonrestorative
6. Perceived need to struggle to overcome inactivity
7. Marked emotional reactivity to feeling fatigued (sadness, frustration, irritability)
8. Difficulty in completing daily tasks attributed to feeling fatigued
9. Perceived problems with short-term memory
10. Post-exertional malaise lasting several hours

The symptoms cause clinically significant distress or impairment in social, occupational, or other important areas of functioning.

There is evidence from the history, physical examination, or laboratory findings that symptoms are a consequence of cancer or cancer-related therapy.

The symptoms are not primarily the consequence of comorbid psychiatric disorders, such as major depression, somatization disorder, somatoform disorder, or delirium.

Adapted from Cella D, Peterman A, Passik S, et al. Progress toward guidelines for the management of fatigue. *Oncol Williston Park N.* 1998;12(11A):369–377.

of validity and reliability. Examples of fatigue measurement tools include the Multidimensional Assessment of Fatigue, the Symptom Distress Scale, the Fatigue Scale, the Fatigue Observation Checklist, and a Visual Analogue Scale for Fatigue. These scales are available for use in research and may be used in the clinical area. In clinical practice, however, a verbal rating scale may be the most efficient. Fatigue severity may be quickly assessed using a "0" (no fatigue) to "10" (extreme fatigue) scale. As with the use of any measure, consistency over time and a specific frame of reference are needed. During each evaluation, the same instructions must be given to the patient. For example, the patient may be asked to rate the level of fatigue for the past 24 hours.

Fatigue, as with any symptom, is not static. Changes take place daily and sometimes hourly in the patient with an advanced illness. As such, fatigue bears repeated evaluation on the part of the health care provider. One patient, noticing the dramatic change in his energy level, remarked, "Have I always been this tired?" He seemed unable to discern whether there had ever been a time when he did not feel overwhelmed by the impact of fatigue. The imperative for palliative care nursing is to consistently take the initiative and ask the patient—and then continue to ask—about fatigue, keeping in mind that the ultimate goal is the patient's comfort. An example of a thorough assessment of the symptom of fatigue is found in Box 1.3, which uses both a subjective and objective framework to ascertain patient fatigue and possible underlying physiologic events that may exacerbate the fatigue.

Management and Treatment

When considering palliative care, the management of fatigue is extremely challenging. By its very definition, palliative care may encompass a prolonged period before death, when a person is still active and physically and socially participating in life, to a few weeks before death, when participatory activity may be minimal. With fatigue interventions, the wishes of the patient and family are paramount. One must consider management in the context of the extent of disease, other symptoms (e.g., pain, nausea, diarrhea), whether palliative treatment is still in process, age and developmental stage, and the emotional "place" of the patient.

Interventions for fatigue have been suggested to occur at two levels: the management of symptoms that contribute to fatigue, and the prevention of additional or secondary fatigue by maintaining a balance between restorative rest and restorative activity. Fatigue interventions have been grouped into two broad categories: pharmacologic interventions and nonpharmacologic interventions.

Pharmacologic Interventions

Pharmacologic approaches to treat fatigue in patients with cancer and chronic progressive diseases have increased. Pharmacologic therapies include antidepressants, psychostimulants, progestional steroids, tumor necrosis factor-α, micronutrients such as L-carnitine, and various other classes of drugs (Table 1.1).[11]

Box 1.3 Primary Fatigue Assessment

Physical examination based on subjective symptom: Perform review of systems. Are there significant comorbidities? Is there anything on examination that could account for the fatigue (recurrence, progression of disease, nerve damage, dehydration, cachexia)?

Medications: Is the patient taking any medications that could contribute to the fatigue (pain or sleep medication, over-the-counter medications, supplements, new medication changes)?

Location: Where on the body is the fatigue located (e.g., upper or lower extremities, all muscles of the body)? Is there mental or attentional fatigue? Is rising from a chair difficult?

Intensity and severity: Does the fatigue interfere with activities (work, role or responsibilities at home, social interaction) or the patient's usual enjoyable activities?

Duration: How long does the fatigue last (minutes, hours, days, time of day)? Has it become chronic (lasting more than 6 months)? What is the pattern (wake up from a night's sleep exhausted, evening fatigue, transient, unpredictable, unfading), and are circadian rhythms affected)? Have there been any changes in duration of fatigue over time?

Aggravating factors: What makes it worse (rest, activity, social interaction, other symptoms, environmental heat, cold, noise)?

Alleviating factors: What relieves it (a good night's rest, food, fluids, caffeine, listening to music, exercise)?

Knowledge of fatigue: Had the patient been prepared for fatigue occurrence? What meaning does the patient assign to the symptom of fatigue (getting worse, disease progression, dying)?

Muscle strength: Perform tests to elicit muscle strength if necessary (Jamar grip dynamometer, nerve conduction studies).

General appearance: Assess general appearance and look for pallor, monotone voice, slowed speech, dull facial expression, stooped shoulders, and weight loss.

Vital signs: Look for anything out of the ordinary to explain fatigue (fever, low blood pressure, irregular heart rate, shortness of breath, weight changes, caloric intake changes).

Laboratory results: Assess oxygenation status (pulse oximeter, hemoglobin, hematocrit), electrolytes, thyroid and adrenal status, white blood cell count, and erythrocyte sedimentation rate.

Level of activity: Has the patient's usual activity changed? How many hours per day in bed or resting?

Affect: What is the mood of the patient (anxious, depressed, sad, apathetic, withdrawn, flat)?

Table 1.1 Pharmacologic Interventions to Relieve Fatigue

Drug Category	Medication
Antidepressants	Paroxetine hydrochloride (Paxil)
	Bupropion (Wellbutrin SR)
Psychostimulants	Methylphenidate (Ritalin)
	Dextroamphetamine
	Modafinil (Provigil)
Progestational steroids	Megestrol acetate or medroxyprogesterone acetate (Megace)
Hemopoietic growth factors	Epoetin alfa (Procrit)
	Darbepoetin alfa (Aranesp)
Tumor necrosis factor-α blockade	Etanercept (Enbrel)
Ongoing medication/other medications and integrative therapies studies	Donepezil (Aricept)
	Levocarnitine (L-carnitine)
	Bisphosphonate
	Ibandronate
	Coenzyme Q_{10}
	American ginseng

Methylphenidate, a psychostimulant, has been shown to improve quality of life when given to depressed, terminally ill patients. It has also been shown to counteract opioid somnolence, enhance the effects of pain medication, improve cognition, and increase patient activity level.[11] Appropriate initial dosing for this drug is 5 to 10 mg orally at breakfast and 5 mg at lunch daily. Some patients require higher doses. Elderly patients may require a downward dose adjustment. However, further research is needed to confirm methylphenidate use in cancer-related fatigue. Dextroamphetamine, a potent central nervous system stimulant, may also be used. This drug is quickly absorbed from the gastrointestinal tract with high concentrations in the brain.

Antidepressants have shown some effectiveness when a patient experiences both fatigue and depression. Corticosteroids, such as prednisone, have been used to increase energy levels at a dose of about 20 to 40 mg/day. Results from one study indicated an increase in activity level when palliative care patients were treated with methylprednisolone. The side effects that may occur with these drugs are always a concern.

Anemia as a result of chemotherapeutic regimens has been very responsive to interventions. Epoetin has been important in increasing hemoglobin levels for some cancer patients to improve quality of life. Doses varying from 10,000 U subcutaneously given three times per week to 40,000 U given once a week have resulted in a similar increase in hemoglobin level. Although results suggest that epoetin has a positive effect on fatigue, there have been safety concerns over possible thromboembolic events. Fewer adverse events are seen when administration was delayed until the hemoglobin was lower than 10 g/dL.

Other drugs and complementary agents have been reported to combat chronic disease-related fatigue, but additional research is warranted.

Nonpharmacologic Interventions

Nonpharmacologic interventions for cancer-related fatigue encompass several disciplines. Historically, nurse clinicians and researchers have been the trailblazers in assessing and managing fatigue in the clinical setting (Table 1.2). Included are patient and staff educational interventions, studies on disrupted sleep patterns, nutritional deficits and their effect on patient quality of life, symptom management, and physical and attentional fatigue.[12]

Table 1.2 Nonpharmacologic Symptom Management Strategies for Fatigue

Problem	Intervention	Rationale
Lack of information or lack of preparation	Explain complex nature of fatigue and importance of communication of fatigue level with health care providers. Explain causes of fatigue in advanced cancer and chronic progressive diseases and evaluate fatigue level with each visit. • Fatigue can increase in advanced disease. • Cancer cells can compete with body for essential nutrients. • Palliative treatments, infection, and fever increase the body's need for energy. • Anxiety, depression, and tension can contribute to fatigue. • Changes in daily schedules or interrupted sleep schedules contribute to fatigue development. Prepare patient for planned activities of daily living and daily events (eating, moving, visitors, health care provider appointments).	Preparatory sensory information reduces anxiety and fatigue. Realistic expectations decrease distress and fatigue.
Disrupted rest and sleep patterns	Evaluate and establish sleep routine. • Evaluate usual sleep pattern, length of uninterrupted sleep, temperature in room, and activity before sleep. • Evaluate eating habits before sleep, medications, and exercise. • Establish and continue regular, routine bedtime and awakening. • Obtain as long sleep sequences as possible, and plan uninterrupted time.	Minimizing time in bed helps patients feel refreshed, avoids fragmented sleep, and strengths circadian rhythm.

(continued)

Table 1.2 (Continued)

Problem	Intervention	Rationale
	• Take short rest periods and naps that do not interfere with night sleep. • Use light sources to cue the body into a consistent sleep rhythm. • Pharmacologic management of insomnia should be used when behavioral and cognitive approaches have been exhausted.	
Deficient nutritional status	Make diet and nutrition recommendations to patient and family • Eat high protein, nutrient dense food to "make every mouthful count." • Use protein supplements to augment diet. • Eat small, frequent meals. • Coordinate time up in chair with meal arrival time. • Socialization may increase oral intake. • Drink 8 glasses per day of fluids, or whatever is tolerated, unless contraindicated. • Consider requesting an appetite stimulant like medroxyprogesterone acetate (Megace).	Increased nutrition will raise energy level. Less energy is needed for digestion with small, frequent meals.
Multi-symptom occurrence	Assess and control symptoms contributing to or coexisting with fatigue, such as pain, sleeplessness, depression, nausea, diarrhea, constipation, electrolyte imbalances, dyspnea, dehydration, infection. Assess for symptoms of anemia and evaluate for the possibility of pharmacologic intervention or transfusion.	Multiple distressing symptoms drain energy and will contribute to marked physical and mental fatigue.
Decreased energy reserves	Plan and schedule activities. • Identify a person to be in charge (fielding questions, answering the phone, organizing meals).	Energy conservation helps the patient to reduce fatigue burden and to efficiently use energy available. Pleasant activities may reduce/relieve mental (attentional) fatigue.

(continued)

Table 1.2 (Continued)

Problem	Intervention	Rationale
	• Adjust method and pace of care and move slowly when providing care.	
	• Prioritize and save energy for the most important events.	
	• Eliminate or postpone noncritical activities.	
	• Learn to listen to your body; if fatigued, rest.	
	Obtain physical therapy consult.	
	• Mild physical therapy may help joint flexibility and prevent pain.	
	• Engage in individually tailored, team-approved exercise or yoga program.	
	Use distraction and restoration.	
	• Encourage activities to restore energy: spending time in natural environment, gardening, listening to music, praying, meditating, engaging in hobbies (art, reading, journaling).	
	• Spend time with family or friends, joining in passive activities (riding in car, watching meal preparation).	

Conclusion

Although fatigue is a complex phenomenon that has been widely studied, there is no universally accepted definition. Fatigue is experienced by individuals with cancer and many other chronic, progressive diseases. It is influenced by many factors, such as age, psychological state, social support, stage of disease, polypharmacy issues, cognitive impairment, and other comorbid conditions. Nurses are challenged to provide ongoing fatigue management education and to support and encourage the patient to actively participate in fatigue management strategies. Patient referral to appropriate members of the treatment team and use of their services are always warranted.

References

1. National Comprehensive Cancer Network. *Practice Guidelines in Oncology Cancer Related Fatigue*. Rockledge, PA: National Comprehensive Cancer Network, 2013. www.nccn.org/index.asp. Accessed December 21, 2014.

2. Radbruch L, Strasser F, Elsner F, et al. Fatigue in palliative care patients: an EAPC approach. *Palliat Med*. 2008;22(1):13–32.

3. Cleeland CS, Bennett GJ, Dantzer R, et al. Are the symptoms of cancer and cancer treatment due to a shared biologic mechanism? A cytokine-immunologic model of cancer symptoms. *Cancer*. 2003;97(11):2919–2925.

4. Schubert C, Hong S, Natarajan L, et al. The association between fatigue and inflammatory marker levels in cancer patients: a quantitative review. *Brain Behav Immun*. 2007;*21*(4):413–427.

5. Woo B, Dibble SL, Piper BF, et al. Differences in fatigue by treatment methods in women with breast cancer. *Oncol Nurs Forum*. 1998;*25*(5):915–920.

6. Luciani A, Jacobsen PB, Extermann M, et al. Fatigue and functional dependence in older cancer patients. *Am J Clin Oncol*. 2008;*31*(5):424–430.

7. So WKW, Marsh G, Ling WM, et al. The symptom cluster of fatigue, pain, anxiety, and depression and the effect on the quality of life of women receiving treatment for breast cancer: a multicenter study. *Oncol Nurs Forum*. 2009;*36*(4):E205–E214.

8. Hauser K, Rybicki L, Walsh D. What's in a name? Word descriptors of cancer-related fatigue. *Palliat Med*. 2010;*24*(7):724–730.

9. De Raaf PJ, de Klerk C, van der Rijt CCD. Elucidating the behavior of physical fatigue and mental fatigue in cancer patients: a review of the literature. *Psychooncology*. 2013;*22*(9):1919–1929.

10. Cella D, Peterman A, Passik S, et al. Progress toward guidelines for the management of fatigue. *Oncol Williston Park N*. 1998;*12*(11A):369–377.

11. Minton O, Richardson A, Sharpe M, et al. A systematic review and meta-analysis of the pharmacological treatment of cancer-related fatigue. *J Natl Cancer Inst*. 2008;*100*(16):1155–1166.

12. Kangas M, Bovbjerg DH, Montgomery GH. Cancer-related fatigue: a systematic and meta-analytic review of non-pharmacological therapies for cancer patients. *Psychol Bull*. 2008;*134*(5):700–741.

Chapter 2

Anorexia and Cachexia

Dorothy Wholihan

Introduction

Management of anorexia-cachexia syndrome (ACS) requires a multimodal, interdisciplinary approach using pharmacologic, nonpharmacologic, and psychosocial interventions.

- *Anorexia* is defined as the reduced or loss of desire to eat[1] and is a symptom that accompanies many common illnesses. In acute events, anorexia usually resolves with resolution of the illness, and any weight lost may be replaced with nutritional supplements or increased intake. Unchecked, anorexia leads to insufficient caloric intake and protein-calorie malnutrition. Weight loss from this starvation phenomenon usually involves loss of fat, rather than muscle tissue. Anorexia is common among patients with advanced cancer and advanced acquired immunodeficiency syndrome (AIDS) but also characterizes the clinical course of patients with other chronic progressive diseases, such as chronic obstructive pulmonary disease, congestive heart failure, and end-stage renal disease.

- Cachexia is a complex syndrome that usually involves anorexia, along with significant weight loss, loss of muscle tissue as well as adipose tissue, and generalized weakness, associated with increased protein catabolism and inflammatory response.[1] *Cachexia* is defined as "a devastating multi-factorial syndrome combining weight loss, depletion of skeletal muscle, anorexia, asthenia, and fatigue"[2] In contrast to the starvation seen in anorexia, in cachexia there is approximately equal loss of fat and muscle, significant loss of bone mineral content, and no response to nutritional supplements or increased intake.

Anorexia-cachexia syndrome is characterized by a variety of signs and symptoms that represent interference with energy intake (e.g., decreased appetite, early satiety, taste changes) and nutritional status (i.e., increased metabolic rate, weight loss, hormonal alterations, muscle and adipose tissue wasting, fatigue and decreased performance status).[1] Whatever the specific disease, the development of ACS poses a significant clinical problem. It is a grave prognostic sign but also has a detrimental effect on quality of life. This syndrome leads to serious physical and functional deficits and can be devastating to self-image, social and family relationships, and spiritual well-being.

Table 2.1 Mechanisms and Effects of Anorexia-Cachexia Syndrome

Mechanisms	Effect
Loss of appetite	Generalized host tissue wasting, nausea or "sick feeling," loss of socialization and pleasure at meals
Reduced voluntary motor activity (fatigue)	Skeletal muscle wasting and inanition (fatigue)
Reduced rate of muscle protein synthesis	Skeletal muscle wasting and asthenia (weakness)
Decreased immune response	Increased susceptibility to infections
Decreased response to therapy	Earlier demise and increased complications of illness

Adapted from Bennami-Baiti N, Davis MP. Cytokines and the cancer anorexia cachexia syndrome. *Am J Hosp Palliat Care.* 2008;25:407–409; and Baldwin C. Nutritional support for malnourished patients with cancer. *Curr Opin Support Palliat Care.* 2011;5:29–36.

Pathophysiology

The basic causes of ACS include the following:
- Decreased food intake
- Metabolic abnormalities
- Actions of pro-inflammatory cytokines
- Systemic inflammation
- Neurohormonal dysregulation
- Tumor by-products
- Catabolic state

There is within some of these mechanisms a mutually reinforcing aspect; for example, anorexia leads to fatigue, fatigue increases anorexia, anorexia increases fatigue, and so on. Table 2.1 summarizes the mechanisms and effects of ACS.[3]

Contributing Factors

Physical Symptoms

A number of physical symptoms of advanced disease may contribute to or cause anorexia, including pain, dysguesia (abnormalities in taste, especially aversion to meat), ageusia (loss of taste), hyperosmia (increased sensitivity to odor), hyposmia (decreased sensitivity to odor), anosmia (absence of sense of smell), stomatitis, dysphagia, odynophagia, dyspnea, hepatomegaly, splenomegaly, gastric compression, delayed emptying, malabsorption, intestinal obstruction, nausea, vomiting, diarrhea, constipation, inanition, asthenia, various infections (see "Oral Issues"), and early satiety. Alcoholism or other substance dependence may also contribute to or cause anorexia. Primary or metastatic disease sites have an effect on appetite, with cancers, such as gastric and pancreatic, having direct effects on organs of alimentation.[1,4]

In general, people who are seriously ill and/or suffering distressing symptoms have a poor appetite. In addition, in cancer, metabolic paraneoplastic syndromes such as hypercalcemia or hyponatremia (syndrome of inappropriate antidiuretic hormone) may also cause anorexia or symptoms such as fatigue that contribute to anorexia. Patients with human immunodeficiency virus (HIV) may also develop primary muscle disease, leading to weight loss.[5,6] Many treatments for chronic diseases have deleterious effects on appetite or result in side effects leading to anorexia and/or weight loss. Each of these should be ruled out as a contributing cause of anorexia and, if present, treated as discussed elsewhere in this book.

Treatment Side Effects

Many interventions used to treat advanced chronic disease have adverse effects on nutritional status. The many medications used to treat HIV/AIDS and its sequelae are an excellent example. Despite the success of highly active antiretroviral therapy in curbing ACS in many patients, the myriad of medications involved in the prevention and treatment of AIDS complications often lead to anorexia and malabsorption themselves, and HIV wasting remains a problem for many.[6] Cytotoxic drugs can be emetogenic, cause taste changes, or cause other gastrointestinal side effects such as oral stomatitis and diarrhea. Radiotherapy can also lead to significant side effects, including nausea, vomiting, diarrhea, xerostomia, and severe fatigue.[5] Among patients with advanced renal disease on dialysis, there is a high prevalence of protein-energy malnutrition.

Psychological and Spiritual Distress

Psychological distress and spiritual distress are often overlooked as causes of anorexia. The physical effects of the illness and/or treatment, coupled with psychological responses (especially anxiety and depression) and spiritual distress, may result in little enthusiasm or energy for preparing or eating food. As weight is lost and energy decreases, changes in self-image occur. Cultural influences must always be considered.

Oral Issues

Special attention should be directed to the oral cavity of patients with advanced disease. The fit of dentures may change with weight loss, or already poorly fitting dentures may not be as well tolerated in advanced disease. Dental pain may be overlooked in the context of terminal illness. Oral and esophageal infections and complications increase with disease progression and immunocompromise. Xerostomia and worsening of tooth decay can occur with radiation therapy. Basic oral hygiene can often be neglected in the setting of advanced illness. Aphthous ulcers, mucositis, candidiasis, aspergillosis, herpes simplex, and bacterial infections cause oral or esophageal pain and, thus, anorexia.

Assessment

Anorexia and weight loss may begin insidiously with only decreased appetite and slight weight loss, which can accompany virtually any illness. As the disease progresses and comorbid conditions increase in number and severity, anorexia and malnutrition increase, and a mutually reinforcing process may emerge. Because ACS is common, and in many cases inevitable, among patients with advanced or terminal illness, identifying specific causes is an extremely challenging task.

Assessment parameters should include appetite, nutritional intake, and basic nutritional status.[7] Appetite is a component of several well-validated tools of global symptom assessment, and simple assessment questions about change in appetite can be transformed into a numerical assessment scale. Intake can be measured retrospectively by recall or prospectively by calorie count. Detailed exploration with appropriate physical examination can identify associated factors (i.e., dysphagia, nausea, oral issues, or pain). Open-ended questions can be helpful in eliciting specific characteristics of the eating problem.

A variety of methods can be used to assess nutritional status, from basic tools such as the Subjective Global Assessment for Nutrition to sophisticated anthropometric and laboratory testing.[7] Common laboratory values may reveal decreased serum albumin, a prognostic indicator of increased morbidity and mortality, as well as changes in several electrolyte and mineral levels.[7]

Perhaps the most important component of assessment in ACS involves the patient's goals of care. Because palliative care encompasses the entire disease continuum, stage of illness and goals of care should be clearly determined before detailed assessment and intervention are planned or initiated. It is imperative to evaluate the degree of suffering or distress experienced as a result of the ACS. A cost−benefit analysis should be undertaken to determine whether a diagnostic workup is valuable in light of the effort, cost, or discomfort it may incur. At some point in the illness, even basic assessments, such as weight, serve only to decrease the patient's quality of life. Assessment parameters are summarized in Box 2.1.

Assessment also includes a psychosocial evaluation, particularly concerning food, determining usual intake patterns, food likes and dislikes, and the meaning of food or eating to the patient and family. Too often, a family member attaches huge significance to nutritional intake and exerts pressure on the patient to increase intake: "If he would just get enough to eat." Giving sustenance is a fundamental means of caring and nurturing, and it is no surprise that the presence of devastating illness often evokes an almost primitive urge to give food. Assessment should also include an evaluation of the patient and family health literacy level, as well as their desire and preferred means of receiving health information.

In some cases, the patient is less troubled than the family by poor nutritional intake. Clinicians should explore the meaning of feeding in the context of the family's cultural and religious background and help to identify other ways in which the family can participate in caring for the patient.

Interventions

The palliative approach to care of the patient with ACS focuses on improving patient comfort and minimizing distress caused by the anorexia and weight

Box 2.1 Assessment Parameters in Anorexia and Cachexia

The patient is likely to report anorexia and/or early satiety.

Weakness (asthenia) and fatigue are present.

Mental status declines, with decreased attention span and ability to concentrate. Depression may increase concurrently.

Inspection/observation may show progressive muscle wasting, loss of strength, and decreased fat. There often is increased total body water, and edema may thus mask some wasting.

Weight may decrease. Weight may reflect nutritional status or fluid accumulation or loss.

Increased weight in the presence of heart disease suggests heart failure.

Triceps skinfold thickness decreases with protein-calorie malnutrition (PCM, skinfold thickness and mid-arm circumference vary with hydration status).

Mid-arm muscle circumference decreases with PCM.

Serum albumin concentrations decrease as nutritional status declines. Albumin has a half-life of 20 days; hence, it is less affected by current intake than other measures.

Other laboratory values associated with anorexia-cachexia syndrome include anemia, increased triglycerides, decreased nitrogen balance, and glucose intolerance.

Adapted from Bennami-Baiti N, Davis MP. Cytokines and the cancer anorexia cachexia syndrome. *Am J Hosp Palliat Care*. 2008;25:407–409; and Leuenberger M, Kurmann S, Stranga, Z. Nutritional screening tools in daily clinical practice: the focus on cancer. *Support Care Cancer*. 2010;18:S17–S27.

loss. Assisting patients and families to adapt to progressive symptoms and alleviating symptoms that may be exacerbating the problem are two foci of interventions. Interventions may combine a variety of approaches, including treatment of secondary (exogenous) causes of anorexia, nutritional support, enteral and parenteral nutrition, pharmacologic management, and psychosocial support.

(Exogenous) Symptom Management

Symptoms that may cause or exacerbate secondary anorexia and weight loss should be evaluated and treated if possible. If anorexia is due to an identifiable problem, such as pain, nausea, fatigue, depression, or taste disorder, appropriate interventions as discussed elsewhere in this book should be instituted. The goal here is to identify and manage potentially correctable problems that contribute to low dietary intake.

Nutritional Support

Oral nutritional support, in an attempt to increase intake or to maximize nutritional content, may be helpful, especially early in the disease process or in specific disease states. The current evidence reveals that improving the quantity and quality of nutrition does not improve lean body mass in patients with cancer.[3] Helping family members understand nutritional needs and limitations in terminal situations is essential. Consultation with a nutrition-ist is usually warranted for the purposes of education and recommendation of appropriate supplements. General guidelines for nutritional interventions include the following:

- The nutritional quality of intake should be evaluated and appropriately modified to improve the quality. Patients who are not moribund may ben-efit emotionally from supplementary sources of protein and calories.

- Culturally appropriate or favored foods should be encouraged. Preserving cultural or social traditions around meals may also be helpful. Families should be encouraged to share mealtime with patients or continue habits such as a glass of wine with meals, if medically appropriate.

- Small meals, on the patient's schedule and according to the taste and whims of the patient, are helpful, at least emotionally, and should be instituted early in the illness so that eating does not become burdensome.

- Foods with different tastes, textures, temperatures, seasonings, degrees of spiciness, degrees of moisture, and colors should be tried, but the fam-ily should be cautioned against overwhelming the patient with a constant parade of foods to try.

- Room-temperature and less spicy foods are preferred by many patients.

- Different liquids should also be tried. Cold, clear liquids are usually well tol-erated and enjoyed, although cultural constraints may exist. For example, patients with illnesses that are classified as "cold" by some Southeast Asians and Latinos are thought to be harmed by taking drinks or foods that are either cold in temperature or thought to have "cold" properties.

- Measures as basic as timing intake may also be instituted. Patients who experience early satiety, for example, should take the most nutritious part of the meal first. Filling fluids without nutritional value (such as carbonated soda) should be avoided at mealtime.

- Oral care must be considered an integral part of nutritional support. Hygiene and management of any oral pain are essential in nutritional support.

- Procedures, treatments, psychological upsets (negative or positive), or other stresses or activities should be limited before meals.

Enteral and Parenteral Nutrition

Enteral feeding (through nasoenteral tube, gastrostomy, or jejunostomy) may be indicated in a small subset of terminally ill patients. Many clinicians postu-late that there exist certain patients with a good functional status and relevant secondary (exogenous) component to their ACS, who may benefit from inva-sive nutritional interventions. Examples include patients with head and neck cancer with severe dysphagia who are undergoing radiation therapy, patients with slow-growing tumors causing bowel obstruction, patients undergoing certain surgeries for upper gastrointestinal malignancies, and those undergo-ing bone marrow transplantation.[8] However, the evidence remains insuffi-cient to recommend specific guidelines for specific populations.

The clinical indications for enteral nutrition in noncancer diagnoses remain controversial, perhaps no more so than in the case of dementia. Although more than 30% of patients with dementia in nursing homes have percutaneous endoscopic gastrostomy tubes, the best available data suggest that tube feeding does not affect quality of life, pressure ulcer formation or healing, aspiration risk, functional capacity, or survival. In these patients, careful hand feeding has been recommended as an alternative. Two nonmalignant conditions warrant consideration of enteral feeding. These include stroke in patients who otherwise have good quality of life and early amyotrophic lateral sclerosis.[9] In general, patients with poor performance status and poor prognosis are at high risk for mortality from gastrostomy.[9] In these patients, comfort feeding should be the primary focus in maintaining quality of life.

The use of parenteral nutrition in ACS has been controversial within the palliative care field, and in nearly all cases, if the patient has a functioning gut, enteral nutrition is preferred over parenteral nutrition because of very limited benefit, less cost, and fewer complications.[9] In palliative care settings, long-term use of parenteral nutrition should be considered only if aligned with goals of care and in those with good underlying functional status and a prognosis of 2 to 3 months and those in whom enteral feeding is not possible. Systematic reviews evaluating the use of total parenteral nutrition in cancer patients found very limited benefit and significantly more infectious, metabolic, and mechanical complications.[4]

Pharmacologic Interventions

Commonly used pharmacologic options with indications and notable side effects are presented in Table 2.2.

Table 2.2 Medications Commonly Used in Anorexia-Cachexia Syndrome

Medication Effects and Common Dosing	Indications	Side Effects and Considerations
Progestational agents, esp. megestrol acetate, 160 to 800 mg/day	Improves appetite, weight gain, and sense of well-being	Thromboembolic events, glucocorticoid effects, gastrointestinal upset, heart failure, menstrual abnormalities, tumor flare
Corticosteroids, e.g., dexamethasone (Decadron), 4 mg/day	Improves appetite and sense of well-being	Immunosuppression, masks infection, hypertension, myopathy, gastrointestinal disturbances, dermal atrophy, increased intracranial pressure, electrolyte imbalances; avoid abrupt cessation
Cannabinoids, e.g., tetrahydrocannabinol (Dronabinol), 5 to 20 mg/day	Increases appetite and decreases anxiety	Somnolence, confusion, dysphoria, especially in elderly patients
Metoclopramide, e.g., 10 mg before meals	Improves gastric emptying, decreases early satiety, improves appetite	Diarrhea, restlessness, fatigue, drowsiness, extrapyramidal side effects

Adapted from Baldwin C. Nutritional support for malnourished patients with cancer. *Curr Opin Support Palliat Care.* 2011;5:29–36.

Box 2.2 Components of a Multimodal Approach to Anorexia-Cachexia Syndrome

1. Early and ongoing determination of goals of care
2. Optimal treatment of underlying disease according to goals of care
3. Prevention, recognition, and prompt treatment of exogenous causes
4. Guidance from nutrition specialists
5. Appropriate pharmacologic interventions
6. Resistance exercise as appropriate
7. Compassionate counseling to patient, family, and significant caregivers with clear consistent and empathetic dialogue

Adapted from Solheim TS, Laird BJA. Evidence base for multimodal therapy in cachexia. *Curr Opin Support Palliat Care.* 2012;6:424–431.

Multimodal Approach

Because of the multidimensional nature of ACS, a multimodal approach is warranted (Box 2.2).[10]

Anorexia and cachexia can have a profound impact on the quality of life of patients, heralding not only physical decline but also significant emotional and social distress. Weight loss negatively affects patient self-esteem but can cause even more distress and anxiety among family and partners. Nurses can play a critical role in assessing patients and family and providing sensitive and culturally appropriate education and support.

Conclusion

Increasingly, ACS is recognized as a serious aspect of advanced or terminal illness. The management of ACS is complicated by numerous obstacles, including lack of clear definition and guidelines, inconsistency in assessment and management strategies, and knowledge deficits about this complex clinical syndrome in health professionals and caregiving families. The challenge is compounded by the interwoven emotional symbolism of food and nurturance. As palliative care providers, we should strive to support, understand, and translate the developing evidence that guides our care. Palliative care nurses are optimally situated to coordinate and drive the necessary multidisciplinary approach to address anorexia and cachexia in advanced, progressive disease.

References

1. Molfino A, Laviano A, Fannelli FP. Contribution of anorexia to tissue wasting in cachexia. *Curr Opin Support Palliat Care.* 2010;4:249–253.
2. Reid J, McKenna H, Fitzsimons D, McCance T. The experience of cancer cachexia: a qualitative study of advanced cancer patients and their family members. *Int J Nurs Stud.* 2009;46:606–616.

3. Bennami-Baiti N, Davis MP. Cytokines and the cancer anorexia cachexia syndrome. *Am J Hosp Palliat Care*. 2008;*25*:407–409.

4. Baldwin C. Nutritional support for malnourished patients with cancer. *Curr Opin Support Palliat Care*. 2011;*5*:29–36.

5. Dodson S, Baracos VE, Jatoi A, et al. Muscle wasting in cancer cachexia: clinical implications, diagnosis, and emerging treatment strategies. *Annu Rev Med*. 2011;*62*:265–279.

6. Thibault R. Cano N, Pichard C. Quantification of lean tissue losses during cancer and HIV infection/AIDS. *Curr Opin Clin Nutr Metab Care*. 2011;*14*:261–267.

7. Leuenberger M, Kurmann S, Stranga Z. Nutritional screening tools in daily clinical practice: the focus on cancer. *Support Care Cancer*. 2010;*18*:S17–S27.

8. Locher JL, Bonner JA, Carroll WR. Prophylactic percutaneous endoscopic gastrostomy tube placement in treatment of head and neck cancer: a comprehensive review and call for evidence-based medicine. *JPEN J Parenter Enteral Nutr*. 2011;*35*:365–374.

9. Dev R, Dalal S, Bruera E. Is there a role for parenteral nutrition or hydration at the end of life? *Curr Opin Support Palliat Care*. 2012;*6*:365–370.

10. Solheim TS, Laird BJA. Evidence base for multimodal therapy in cachexia. *Curr Opin Support Palliat Care*. 2012;*6*:424–431.

Chapter 3

Artificial Nutrition and Hydration

Michelle S. Gabriel and Jennifer A. Tschanz

Introduction

In the context of providing palliative care, decisions to initiate or withhold and withdraw the interventions of artificial nutrition and hydration (ANH) can be challenging for the patient, the family, and members of the health care team. In many cultures, providing food and fluids is synonymous with caring, hope, and comfort.[1] Decreased appetite or inability to tolerate or enjoy food and fluids is often a hallmark of the terminal phase of an illness. Individuals and their families may ask for ANH to address a variety of situations (e.g., fears of starvation, weight loss, and dehydration).

As with any palliative care intervention, the nurse needs to understand the patient's illness trajectory and patient and family goals of care, which can be influenced by a person's culture or religion. The nurse also needs to be familiar with the current evidence for ANH in patients with advanced illness because nurses often participate in conversations regarding treatment options and have a critical role in supporting the patient in identifying interventions that best meet their goals.

Artificial Nutrition

Artificial nutrition is an intervention to address malnutrition, which has been linked to poorer outcomes, such as increased mortality, infections, and pressure ulcers. Malnutrition occurs when the body does not get the nutrients it needs. Causes of malnutrition include an inadequate diet, mechanical issues with digestion or absorption of nutrients, and specific medical conditions.[2] In patients with advanced chronic disease or terminal illness, specific causes for malnutrition may result from anorexia, cachexia, and physiologic issues. Anorexia manifests with a decrease in appetite, which can lead to a loss of fat tissue. The weight loss that results can be reversible depending on the underlying causes. Many patients with advanced illness experience anorexia. Cancer cachexia is a multifactorial syndrome in which there is loss of skeletal muscle that cannot be completely reversed by nutritional support, resulting in a negative impact on functional status.[2] Mechanical issues include malignant bowel obstruction and dysphagia.

Methods of Administration

Artificial nutrition is the delivery of nutrients to an individual that bypasses the oral route.[2] It can be administered enterally or parenterally.

- Methods to provide *enteral nutrition*, which accesses the body's gastrointestinal tract, consist of nasogastric, nasointestinal, percutaneous gastrostomy (PEG), or jejunostomy access, with PEG being the preferred method of access for long-term feeding.

- *Parenteral nutrition*, which instills nutrients directly into the circulatory system, can be delivered through a peripheral vein, using peripheral parenteral nutrition (PPN), or through a central line, using total parenteral nutrition (TPN).

Benefits and Burdens

Although the benefits of artificial nutrition are clearer in patients who are expected to recover, they are not as clear in patients who have advanced chronic illness or who are terminally ill. The expected benefits include improving a patient's nutritional status to alleviate distressing symptoms resulting from malnutrition; however, artificial nutrition in the palliative care setting does not always have a positive impact. For patients with amyotrophic lateral sclerosis (ALS), there are guidelines recommending the use and timing of artificial nutrition because malnutrition and weight loss are prognosticators for survival.[3] In patients with cancers of the oropharynx or esophagus, artificial nutrition may be appropriate earlier in the disease trajectory, especially when the cause of malnutrition is directly related to the inability to maintain intake because of mechanical blockages and acute treatment effects (e.g., mucositis secondary to chemoradiation).[4]

Although there may be some benefit in certain populations with end-stage diseases, enteral and parenteral feedings are interventions with the potential for associated morbidity and increased suffering. Potential complications from the administration of artificial nutrition are listed in Table 3.1. Potential additional burdens include: complications from tube placement, increased risk of infection or skin excoriation around the tube, and use of mechanical or pharmacologic restraints to preserve access.

Factors Associated With Considering Artificial Nutrition

- *Malnutrition, anorexia, and cachexia:* In many end-stage diseases, weight loss due to malnutrition, anorexia, or cachexia is a common occurrence. In the terminal phase of diseases such as cancer, artificial nutrition may not be metabolized in a way that would reverse the effects, and the intervention for palliative purposes is rarely recommended.

- *Dysphagia:* When a patient has difficulty swallowing, artificial nutrition may be considered to ensure that the patient receives adequate nutrition or to reduce the risk for aspiration pneumonia. In certain disease states, such as ALS and dementia, it is a matter of when, not if, dysphagia will occur. Providers may consider initiating enteral feeds to reduce the risk for

Table 3.1 Potential Complications of Enteral Support

Complication	Symptom	Cause
Aspiration	Coughing	Excess residual
	Fever	Large-bore tube
Diarrhea	Watery stool	Hyperosmotic solution
		Rapid infusion
		Lactose intolerance
Constipation	Hard, infrequent stools	Inadequate fluid
		Inadequate fiber
Dumping syndrome	Dizziness	High volume
		Hyperosmotic fluids

aspiration pneumonia due to "food going down the wrong way"; however, recent studies have shown that enteral nutrition does not reduce, and may increase, the risk for aspiration pneumonia.

- *Hunger:* Families often express concern about their loved one experiencing hunger, or fears about their loved one starving at end of life, yet patients will often deny sensations of hunger in the terminal phase. In advanced cancer and dementia, hunger is not a symptom often experienced because of the disease process.
- *Pressure ulcers:* Patients who are malnourished are at increased risk for pressure ulcers, yet at the end of life, there is no evidence to support the use of artificial nutrition to treat or prevent pressure ulcers.[5]
- *Survival time:* There is no compelling evidence that artificial nutrition increases the survival of patients with end-stage diseases.
- *Quality of life:* There have not been many studies that specifically measure quality of life for patients with end-stage illness receiving artificial nutrition.

Summary

Artificial nutrition has been shown to have a positive impact on survival and nutritional parameters in certain populations, such as earlier in the disease trajectory in patients with ALS or some cancers. However, there is not enough evidence to support a specific recommendation on when or if, in a palliative care population, it is best to use artificial nutrition. The individual patient's condition, along with the goals of care, needs to be considered to best determine the benefit of employing artificial nutrition compared with the burdens of the intervention.

Hydration

Hydration is an intervention used to address end-of-life situations such as fluid deficits and altered mental status secondary to medication toxicities. Symptoms may include thirst, anorexia, nausea and vomiting, fatigue, and irritability. Physical findings may include lethargy, confusion, muscle twitching, and hyperreflexia. Physical examination will reveal diminished skin turgor and capillary refill as well as orthostatic hypotension. Patients with advanced illness experiencing anorexia may also experience a loss of interest in drinking. During the terminal phase, fluid deficits, similar to malnutrition, may result from anorexia, early satiety, nausea and vomiting, bowel obstruction, dysphagia, and cognitive impairment.

Some patients and families believe that decreased oral intake and the ensuing dehydration causes suffering. Patients and families are concerned that dehydration may precipitate symptoms of delirium, confusion, myoclonus, somnolence, fatigue, neuromuscular irritability, restlessness, thirst, hunger, and constipation, especially in the presence of opioids, benzodiazepines, and neuroleptics. There is limited information regarding the effects of hydration in addressing these symptoms.

When considering hydration, it is important to consider where the patient is on the disease trajectory (e.g., acutely ill or in the dying phase) to help establish goals of care.[6] Hydration can be used for the temporary relief of symptoms of fluid loss, such as nausea, vomiting, diarrhea, and fevers; to decrease fatigue; to improve mental cognition status associated with medication toxicities; and in respect of cultural and familial beliefs.

Methods of Administration

Various alternative routes to oral administration can meet the goals of care and wishes of the patient and family. Standard methods for replacement of fluids, similar to nutrition, can be achieved by the use of enteral feeding tubes and parenteral methods, such as subcutaneous or intravenous infusion.

- *Intravenous access* requires a competent vein. Clinicians may use permanent access devices if they have previously been placed or if ongoing hydration is anticipated.

- *Hypodermoclysis* is the subcutaneous infusion of isotonic solution. It does not require special access devices and can be used for patients who have poor venous access for intravenous placement. The absorption of the subcutaneous fluids has been found to be comparable with absorption of intravenous fluids when administered appropriately.[6]

- *Proctoclysis* is used to administer water or saline into the gastrointestinal tract through the rectum using a nasogastric tube. Researchers have found proctoclysis to be safe and economical, but there has been cultural and social reluctance to accept this mode of administration.[7]

There is no consensus regarding the volume or type of fluid replacement. Risks and burdens must be considered (Table 3.2).

Benefits and Burdens

The decision for hydration needs to include an evaluation of goals of care, discussion of the risks and benefits, and timely re-evaluation to determine whether goals or symptoms are improving or worsening.[6,7]

- Risks for overhydration—as evidenced by worsening fluid retention, signs of increased shortness of breath, increased emotional distress, or change in mental status—must be monitored.

Table 3.2 Potential Complications of Routes for Artificial Hydration

Intravenous: Peripheral	Intravenous: Central	Subcutaneous: Hypodermoclysis
Pain	Sepsis	Pain
Short duration of access	Hemothorax	Infection
Infection	Pneumothorax	Third spacing
Phlebitis	Central vein thrombosis	Tissue sloughing
	Catheter fragment thrombosis	Local bleeding
	Air embolus	
	Brachial plexus injury	
	Arterial laceration	

- Advantages of not providing artificial hydration can include reduced urine output, leading to reduced incontinence and need for catheterization; reduction of gastrointestinal secretions, leading to decreased incidence of vomiting; and decreased respiratory tract secretions, leading to decreased cough and need for suction.

- Factors arguing against initiating hydration include increasing the incidence of pulmonary edema, peripheral edema, increased respiratory tract secretions, cough, and ascites.

- Starting intravenous hydration can cause pain, be distressing, restrict mobility, hinder family contact, and increase the use of restraints.

Review of the Literature

- *Dehydration and fluid retention:* Dehydration can cause unpleasant symptoms, such as confusion and restlessness, in non–terminally ill patients. These problems are common in dying people. There is limited research regarding the effect of hydration on alleviating dehydration at the end of life.

- *Thirst and dry mouth:* Thirst is thought to be a nonspecific symptom of dehydration. Routine care, defined as offering food and fluids, administering ice chips, and providing mouth care, helps to alleviate these symptoms. Dry mouth is treated with an intensive, every-2-hour schedule of mouth care, including hygiene, lip lubrication, and ice chips or popsicles. Elimination of medications that cause dry mouth, such as tricyclic antidepressants and antihistamines, should be considered. Sometimes, drugs that contribute to these symptoms are being administered to palliate other symptoms, such as the opioids for pain and anticholinergics, to minimize oral secretions. Mouth breathing can also contribute to dry mouth. *Candida* infection, a frequent cause of dry mouth, can be treated. Agents such as pilocarpine (Salagen) can be used to increase salivation.

- *Delirium, confusion, agitation:* Delirium can be caused by multiple factors, including end-organ failure, dehydration, and medications. Symptoms of delirium can be distressful for patients and families. In advanced cancer patients, no significant difference in delirium and agitation was noted between patients receiving more hydration than less hydration. If delirium is related to the accumulation of opioids, interventions to decrease or rotate opioids and to increase hydration are believed to control symptoms of hyperactive delirium, such as agitation and hallucinations of opioid-induced neurotoxicity, by assisting with the clearance of toxic opioid metabolites.

- *Myoclonus:* Myoclonus, or involuntary contractions of muscles, is commonly associated with chronic opioid use at the end of life. It has also been reported in cancer patients without opioid use who are experiencing decreased oral intake. There is limited and mixed information regarding the effects of hydration on myoclonus, depending on patient setting.

- *Survival benefit:* There is limited research regarding the survival benefit of hydration. Two studies noted that hydration provided no survival benefit for terminally ill cancer patients with short prognosis.

- *Quality of life:* There is limited research regarding the impact of hydration on quality of life in terminally ill patients.

Summary

Parenteral hydration has been found to be effective in temporary, short-term situations to alleviate symptoms related to dehydration and improve mental cognition. In the palliative care setting, research does not support that parenteral hydration improves signs of dehydration, survival, or quality of life. In the setting of delirium related to opioid toxicity, there is mixed evidence supporting hydration and possible opioid rotation to improve delirium symptoms. When deciding to initiate or stop hydration, it is important to assess goals of care, risks and benefits, and the patient's preferences.

Review of Position Statements and Guidelines

Many professional organizations have published position statements or guidelines on the use of ANH. Common themes across these documents include the following:

- ANH is an intervention that should be evaluated by the patient, family, and care team considering its benefits and burdens.

Table 3.3 Disease-Specific Guidelines for Artificial Nutrition and Hydration

Advanced dementia	• Feeding tubes are not recommended. • Oral feedings are enhanced by improving the environment and supporting patient-centered approaches.
End-stage cancer	• Use of nutritional support for terminally ill cancer patients is not usually indicated.
Amyotrophic lateral sclerosis	• Early insertion of a feeding tube is recommended if enteral feeding is determined to be an appropriate intervention.

- ANH is considered a medical intervention that can be refused, withheld, or withdrawn based on the patient's clinical condition and goals of care.
- Decisions about ANH need to reflect the patient and family's values, beliefs, and culture.

In addition to general position statements regarding ANH, disease specific recommendations are summarized in Table 3.3.

Role of Religion and Culture

Decisions about the initiation or withholding and withdrawing of ANH are complex.[8,9] To deliver patient-centered care, nurses must recognize the role that religious or spiritual beliefs and culture, including race and ethnicity, play on patient and family values of food and fluids. Understanding these factors and encouraging a dialog about patient values will enable nurses to respect patient autonomy and engage in a dialogue about how to meet patient needs regarding nutrition and hydration. In reviewing common beliefs of various religious traditions and cultures, it is important to remember that not everyone of a particular faith or a particular culture will have the same beliefs, so nurses should inquire as to how much influence a patient's faith or culture has on his or her beliefs regarding ANH.

Major religions have varying beliefs specific to the use of life-sustaining therapies such as ANH. Even within religions, there can be varying opinions or interpretations of religious law to guide decisions about whether to initiate or withdraw ANH.[9-13] Table 3.4 summarizes beliefs by selected religious traditions specific to ANH.

Table 3.4 Religious Beliefs Regarding Artificial Nutrition and Hydration	
Religious Faith	**Beliefs**
Buddhism	• Buddhists believe that all beings suffer. • The main focus at end of life is on spiritual comfort. • There is less focus on extending life through artificial nutrition and hydration (ANH) and other interventions.
Catholicism	• The current position (as of 2011) focuses on "life prolongation based on fundamental human dignity." • Some within the church assert that ANH is not considered a medical technology but rather an ordinary measure to preserve life. • Others feel that ANH should be evaluated using the proportionate/disproportionate framework (ordinary versus extraordinary) on an individual basis. • Catholic health care facilities are obligated to offer food and fluids regardless of disease state. • ANH can be considered extraordinary in conditions in which the underlying disease would be the cause of death, not the withholding of ANH.

(continued)

Table 3.4 (Continued)	
Religious Faith	**Beliefs**
Hinduism	• Withholding or withdrawal of ANH at the very end of life is acceptable.
	• Some Hindus fast to prepare for death.
Islam	• "Guiding purpose of Islamic law is to protect and preserve religion, life, progeny, intellect, and wealth."
	• Islamic rules regarding care for terminally ill are based on the principle that one should prevent or avoid injury or harm.
	• Islamic law permits withdrawal of ANH and allowing the disease to take its natural course.
	• There can be various beliefs among Muslims, so it is necessary to know the individual patient's values.
	• "Islamic law states that palliative care should not shorten a patient's life, but futile treatment is not justified."
	• "Islamic law forbids passively or actively causing death."
	• Nutritional support is considered basic care and not medical treatment, leading to a duty to feed patients who are no longer able to feed themselves.
	• There is varied opinion among different Islamic communities regarding withdrawing and withholding ANH.
Judaism	• Provision of food and fluids is considered an ordinary measure, not extraordinary.
	• Withholding food and fluids is not consistent with Jewish law.
	• Administration of food and fluids, even through an intravenous or feeding tube, is not considered to be artificial.
	• "The religious authorities hold that [ANH] are ordinary supportive measures rather than heroic."
	• "Terminal dehydration, hospice without provision of ANH, and withdrawing or withholding ANH is not considered aligned with Jewish teaching unless there is proof of 'goses' (less than 72 hours until death) and futility of intervention under any denomination of Judaism."
	• "While the [Israeli] law respects the right of a competent dying patient to refuse nutrition and hydration, it introduces a legal requirement to persuade 'the use of oxygen, nutrition and hydration,' even by artificial means."
Protestantism	• There is diversity in positions regarding ANH across denominations
	• Protestants commonly believe that interventions such as ANH that allow time for repentance may outweigh other burdens of treatment.
Adapted from references 9 to 13.	

perspectives of ANH. Studies have shown variance associated with race in the use of tube feedings, with whites having lower rates than people of other cultural backgrounds. Although there is not a large body of research on how differing religious and cultural backgrounds influence individual preferences for ANH, there are resources that nurses can access to learn information needed to initiate a conversation with a patient on this issue. Whether it is through position statements from religious organizations or talking to leaders within a particular faith tradition or ethnic community, nurses can seek to understand how these factors play a role in each specific situation with the patient for whom they are caring.

Engaging in Conversations About Artificial Nutrition and Hydration

In working with palliative care and terminally ill patients, nurses play a critical role in exploring a patient's values and hopes to ensure that care related to the provision of food and fluids is patient centered. Because decisions about ANH are complex, nurses have multiple responsibilities. Nurses need to self-reflect on their own personal values, similarly influenced by religious and cultural factors as well as clinical experience. Just as continuing education and experience help nurses to develop clinical skills and understanding, further and continued ethics education may be helpful to sharpen skills in reasoning through the ANH debate to better support patients and families in the decision-making process. Position statements by established professional nursing and medical organizations and outcomes of landmark legal decisions regarding ANH can provide a foundation for how nurses and the health care team approach conversations with the family about ANH.

Initiating and Withdrawing or Withholding Artificial Nutrition and Hydration

If the decision is made to initiate ANH in a patient to meet the goals of care, the nurse has a responsibility to continually assess the patient's condition, evaluating the impact of the intervention on symptoms and the patient's responses to treatment. ANH can be offered as a time-limited trial to determine whether the patient experiences any benefits from the intervention compared with burdens. Because artificial nutrition is often instituted during an acute event while in the hospital, nurses can inquire about previous medical history or expressed wishes and promote conversations that look at the bigger picture beyond the acute admission.[8] Nurses in any setting can inform patients and families early in the disease continuum of the progression of the illness, and ensure that wishes are elicited and documented by the health care team regarding ANH. The nurse needs to facilitate ongoing conversations about ANH to ensure that the role of this therapy continues to meet patient and family goals without excessive burden.

If the decision is made to either withdraw or withhold ANH, the nurse can provide emotional support and assurances that the patient's dignity will be respected with comfort care. If unable to support a patient or family's decision regarding ANH for religious or personal reasons, it is the responsibility of the nurse to request a change in assignment and for the health care system to ensure that a nurse comfortable in these situations can provide patient-centered care when ANH is being withheld or withdrawn.

Conclusion

The provision of food and fluids is synonymous with caring across many cultures. When a patient experiences a decreased desire to eat or drink as part of the end stage of illness, the patient, along with the family, may struggle and seek interventions to extend life, reduce the impact of possible symptoms such as hunger or dehydration, or fulfill a religious or cultural need at the end of life. Nurses need to understand the factors, such as religion and culture, that influence a patient's preferences. Nurses need to provide accurate and complete information about the benefits and burdens of ANH. In doing so, nurses will ensure that decisions to initiate, withhold, or withdraw ANH will be patient centered.

References

1. Cohen MZ, Torres-Vigil I, Burbach BE, et al. The meaning of parenteral hydration to family caregivers and patients with advanced cancer receiving hospice care. *J Pain Symptom Manage.* 2012;43(5):855–865.

2. Hospice and Palliative Nurses Association. Artificial nutrition and hydration in advanced illness. *J Hosp Palliat Nurs.* 2012;14(3):173–176.

3. Morassutti I, Giometto M, Baruffi C, et al. Nutritional intervention for amyotrophic lateral sclerosis. *Minerva Gastroenterol Dietol.* 2012;58(3)253–260.

4. Pfister DV, Ang K, Brizel DM, et al. NCCN clinical practice guidelines in oncology (NCCN Guidelines®): Head and neck cancers (Version 2.2013). National Comprehensive Cancer Network Web site. http://www.nccn.org/professionals/physician_gls/pdf/head-and-neck.pdf. May 29, 2013. Accessed July 21, 2013.

5. Teno JM, Gozalo P, Mitchell SL, et al. Feeding tubes and the prevention or healing of pressure ulcers. *Arch Intern Med.* 2012;172(9):697–701.

6. Dalal S, Del Fabbro E, Bruera E. Is there a role for hydration at the end of life? *Curr Opin Support Palliat Care.* 2009;3(1):72–78.

7. Nakajima N, Hata Y, Kusumuto K. A clinical study on the influence of hydration volume on the signs of terminally ill cancer patients with abdominal malignancies. *J Palliat Med.* 2013;16(2):185–189.

8. Geppert CM, Andrews MR, Druyan ME. Ethical issues in artificial nutrition and hydration: a review. *J Parenter Enteral Nutr.* 2010;34(1):79–88.

9. Brody H, Hermer LD, Scott LD, et al. Artificial nutrition and hydration: the evolution of ethics, evidence, and policy. *J Gen Intern Med.* 2011;26(9):1053–1058.

10. Bradley CT. Roman Catholic doctrine guiding end-of-life care: a summary of the recent discourse. *J Palliat Med.* 2009;12(4):373–377.

11. Alsolamy S. Islamic views on artificial nutrition and hydration in terminally ill patients. *Bioethics* 2014;*28*(2):96–99.

12. Rosner F, Abramson N. Fluids and nutrition: perspectives from Jewish Law (Halachah). *South Med J.* 2009;*102*(3):248–250.

13. Ravitsky V. A Jewish perspective on the refusal of life-sustaining therapies: culture as shaping bioethical discourse. *Am J Bioeth.* 2009;*9*(4):60–62.

Chapter 4

Urinary Tract Disorders

Mikel Gray and Terran Sims

Introduction

Urinary system disorders may be directly attributable to a malignancy, systemic disease, or a specific treatment such as radiation or chemotherapy. In many ways, the techniques used for management of urinary symptoms are similar to those used for patients in any care setting. However, in contrast to traditional interventions, the evaluation and management of urinary tract symptoms in the palliative care setting are influenced by considerations of the goals of care and closeness to death.

Lower Urinary Tract Disorders

Urinary Incontinence

Urinary incontinence (UI) is defined as the uncontrolled loss of urine of sufficient magnitude to create a problem.[1] It can be divided into two types: transient (acute) and chronic, based on onset and underlying etiology. Factors resulting in transient UI clearly contribute to urinary leakage, but they often arise from outside the lower urinary tract. Therefore, treatment of transient UI is typically aimed at the contributing factor, rather than the urinary system itself. Several conditions associated with transient UI are commonly encountered when caring for patients in a palliative care setting; they include delirium, urinary tract infection, adverse side effects of various drugs, restricted mobility, and severe constipation or stool impaction (Table 4.1).

Chronic UI is subdivided into types according to its presenting symptoms or underlying pathophysiology. Stress UI occurs when physical stress (exertion) causes urine loss in the absence of a detrusor contraction. Intrinsic sphincter deficiency occurs when the nerves or muscles necessary for sphincter closure are denervated or damaged. Box 4.1 lists conditions that are likely to cause intrinsic sphincter deficiency in patients receiving palliative care.

Urge UI occurs when overactive detrusor contractions produce urinary leakage (Table 4.2). Urge UI is part of a larger symptom syndrome called *overactive bladder*. Overactive bladder is characterized by urgency (a sudden desire to urinate that is difficult to defer), and it is typically associated with daytime voiding frequency (more than every 2 hours) and nocturia (≥3 episodes per night).

Table 4.1 Factors Associated With Urinary Incontinence in the Patient Receiving Palliative Care

Associated Factor	Effect on Continence
Delirium, confusion	Patient's reduced ability to recognize and respond to cues to urinate results in daytime or nighttime urinary incontinence (UI) episodes.
Urinary tract infection	Infection may exacerbate or create transient UI, especially in patients with history of UI or overactive bladder dysfunction.
Various drugs	Multiple classes of drugs predispose vulnerable patients to UI; diuretics increase urine production, potentially increasing frequency of and risk for overactive detrusor contractions; antidepressants, sedatives, sleeping medications, or opioid analgesics may reduce the individual's ability to detect or respond to cues to toilet.
Excessive urine output	Polyuria associated with diabetes mellitus, diabetes insipidus, chronic venous disease, chronic heart failure, renal insufficiency, or high-volume fluid intake increases urine production, potentially increasing voiding frequency and risk for overactive detrusor contractions.
Restricted mobility	Immobility, secondary to pain to as a direct result of a disease process affecting neuromuscular function, impairs the individual's ability to respond to cues to toilet and to access toilet facilities.
Constipation or stool impaction	Exact mechanism is unknown; distention of the rectal vault may reduce bladder capacity and cause functional obstruction by reflex increase in pelvic floor muscle tone as the vault fills with stool.

Box 4.1 Causes of Intrinsic Sphincter Deficiency in the Patient Receiving Palliative Care

Urethral Surgery

Radical prostatectomy
Transurethral prostatectomy
Cryosurgery
Suburethral sling surgery for stress urinary incontinence in women

Surgical Procedures Indirectly Affecting the Urethra Through Local Denervation

Abdominoperineal resection
Pelvic exenteration
Radical hysterectomy

Neurologic Lesions of the Lower Spine

Primary or metastatic tumors of the sacral spine
Pathologic fracture of the sacral spinal column
Multiple sclerosis
Tertiary syphilis

Table 4.2 Conditions Associated With Detrusor Overactivity in the Patient Receiving Palliative Care

Condition	Disorder
Neurologic lesions above the brainstem micturition center	Overactive bladder, with or without urge urinary incontinence (UI)
	Posterior fossa tumors causing intracranial pressure increased
Primary or metastatic tumors of the spinal segments	Cerebrovascular accident (stroke)
	Diseases affecting the brain, including multiple sclerosis, AIDS
Neurologic lesions below the brainstem micturition center but above sacral spinal segments	Reflex UI with vesicosphincter dyssynergia
	Primary or metastatic tumors of the spinal cord
	Tumors causing spinal cord compression because of their effects on the spinal column
	Systemic diseases directly affecting the spinal cord, including advanced-stage AIDS, transverse myelitis, Guillain-Barré syndrome
Inflammation of the bladder	Overactive bladder, with or without urge UI
	Primary bladder tumors, including papillary tumors or carcinoma in situ
	Bladder calculi (stones)
	Radiation cystitis, including brachytherapy
	Chemotherapy-induced cystitis
Bladder outlet obstruction	Overactive bladder, usually without urge UI
	Prostatic carcinoma
	Urethral cancers
	Pelvic tumors causing urethral compression

Reflex UI, in contrast, is caused by a neurologic lesion below the brainstem micturition center. It is characterized by diminished or absent sensations of bladder filling, neurogenic overactive detrusor contractions associated with urinary leakage, and a loss of coordination between the detrusor and sphincter muscles (detrusor-sphincter dyssynergia).

Functional UI occurs when long-standing deficits in mobility, dexterity, or cognition cause or contribute to urinary leakage. A variety of conditions may produce functional UI in the patient receiving palliative care. For example, neurologic deficits or pain may reduce the patient's ability to reach the toilet in a timely fashion. Cognitive deficits caused by malignancies or diseases of the brain may predispose the patient to functional UI. In addition, sedative or analgesic medications may reduce awareness of bladder fullness and the need to urinate, particularly in the patient who experiences nocturia.

Extraurethral UI occurs when a fistula creates an opening between the bladder and the vagina or skin, allowing urine to bypass the urethral sphincter. Within the context of palliative care, fistulas are usually caused by invasive pelvic or gynecologic malignancies, extensive pelvic surgery, or radiation treatment.

Bladder Spasm

Bladder spasm may be defined as a painful contraction of the bladder, usually caused by an overactive detrusor contraction against a closed or partially blocked bladder outlet. Patients with bladder outlet obstruction due to a urologic malignancy obstructing the bladder outlet or secondary blockage from a tumor outside the urinary tract are at risk for bladder spasm. Foreign objects within the urinary tract, such as indwelling urinary catheters or ureteral stents, are also associated with an increased risk for bladder spasm.[2]

Assessment and Management of Bothersome Lower Urinary Tract Symptoms

Assessment

The results of a focused history, physical assessment, urinalysis, and bladder log are essential for the evaluation of UI in the patient receiving palliative care. Urine culture and sensitivity testing, blood tests, urodynamic evaluation, or imaging studies also may be completed in specific cases. The history focuses on the duration of the problem and the probable cause of bothersome lower urinary tract symptoms (LUTS).

- Transient UI is typically characterized by a sudden occurrence of urinary leakage or an acute exacerbation of preexisting symptoms. These symptoms are typically similar to those of urge or stress UI.

- Stress UI is characterized by urine loss occurring with physical exertion or a sudden increase in abdominal pressure caused by coughing or sneezing. It occurs in the absence of a precipitous and strong urge to urinate.

- Reflex UI is suspected in the patient who experiences a paralyzing neurologic lesion that affects spinal segments below the brainstem and above S2. The patient frequently reports periodic urination with little or no warning and little or no associated urgency. The urinary stream may be intermittent (stuttering), and the patient may perceive a sensation of incomplete bladder emptying or report additional urinary leakage soon after completion of micturition.

- Functional UI is suspected when a general evaluation of the patient reveals significant limitations in mobility, dexterity, or cognition.

Continuous urinary leakage that is not associated with physical exertion raises the suspicion of extraurethral UI associated with a fistula, but it is also associated with severe stress UI caused by intrinsic sphincter deficiency. Bladder spasms are diagnosed when a patient reports painful episodes localized to the suprapubic or lower abdomen. These pains are usually characterized by a sudden onset and are described as stabbing, cramping, or colicky. They are often associated with urgency and may produce bypassing of urine around an indwelling urinary catheter or urethral leakage if a suprapubic catheter is in place.

Physical Examination

A focused physical examination provides additional evidence concerning the UI type and its severity. A general examination is used to evaluate the presence of functional UI and to determine the influence of functional limitations on other types of UI. A pelvic examination is completed to assess perineal skin integrity, to identify the presence of obvious fistulas or severe sphincter incompetence, and to evaluate local neurologic function. Altered skin integrity, particularly if accompanied by a monilial rash or incontinence-associated dermatitis, may occur, especially in patents with double fecal and urinary incontinence.[3]

Bladder Log

A bladder log (a written record of the timing of urination, voided volume, timing of UI episodes, and fluid intake) is useful because it allows a semiquantitative analysis of the patterns of urinary elimination, UI, and associated symptoms. It can also be used to assess fluid intake or the patient's response to prompted voiding. The patient is taught to record the time of voluntary urination, episodes of incontinence and associated factors (urgency, physical activity), and type and amount of fluids consumed. Recording fluid intake allows the nurse to calculate the cumulative volume of fluids consumed each day, as well as the proportion of fluids containing caffeine or alcohol—substances that exacerbate bothersome LUTS.

Laboratory Evaluation

Urinalysis serves several useful purposes in the evaluation of the patient with UI. The presence of nitrites and leukocytes on dipstick analysis or bacteriuria and pyuria on microscopic analysis may indicate a clinically relevant urinary tract infection. Blood in the urine may coexist with a urinary tract infection, or it may indicate significant hematuria demanding prompt management. In the patient receiving palliative care, glucosuria may indicate poorly controlled diabetes mellitus causing osmotic diuresis and subsequent UI. In contrast, a low specific gravity may indicate diabetes mellitus or excessive fluid intake from oral or parenteral sources.

A urine culture and sensitivity analysis is obtained if the urinalysis reveals bacteriuria and pyuria, and an endoscopy is indicated if significant hematuria is present without an obvious explanation. Urodynamic testing is indicated in selected patients after transient UI is excluded and when simpler examinations have failed to establish an accurate diagnosis leading to an effective plan for management.

Management of Urinary Incontinence

The management of UI is based on its type, the desires of the patient and family, and the presence of complicating factors. Transient UI is managed by addressing its underlying cause.

- Acute delirium is managed by treating the underlying infection of disease causing the delirium, if feasible.

- A urinary tract infection is treated with sensitivity-driven antibiotics.
- Medication regimens are altered as feasible if they produce or exacerbate UI.
- Fecal impaction must be relieved and constipation aggressively managed. After initial disimpaction, a scheduled elimination program is frequently indicated

A number of techniques are used to manage chronic or established UI. Every patient should be counseled about lifestyle alterations that may alleviate or occasionally relieve UI and associated LUTS.

- Patients are advised to avoid routinely restricting fluid intake to reduce UI because this strategy only increases the risk for constipation and concentrates the urine, irritating the bladder wall. Instead, they should be counseled to obtain the recommended daily allowance for fluids (1.5 to 2.3 liters in adults; 1.2 to 2.3 liters in adults >70 years of age), to sip fluids throughout the day, and to avoid intake of large volumes of fluids over a brief period.
- Patients may also be taught to reduce or avoid bladder irritants that increase urine production or stimulate increased detrusor muscle tone, including caffeine and alcohol, depending on the goals of care and the short-term prognosis.

Containment devices may be used to provide protection while treatments designed to address underlying UI are undertaken, or they may be used for added protection if these interventions improve but fail to eradicate urine loss. Women and men should be counseled about the disadvantages of using home products and feminine hygiene pads when attempting to contain urine. As an alternative, patients should be advised about products specifically designed for UI, including disposable and reusable products, inserted pads, and containment briefs.

If the patient experiences primarily stress UI, the initial management is with behavioral methods, often combined with use of absorptive products. Pelvic floor muscle training is strongly recommended for mild to moderate stress UI,[4] but its applicability in the palliative care setting is limited. Instead, the patient may be taught a maneuver called the "knack" (Box 4.2).

Medications also may be used to treat stress UI in selected cases. Table 4.3 describes pharmacologic options for managing overactive bladder and urge UI and related nursing considerations.[5]

Patients whose LUTS are not managed adequately by behavioral methods should be counseled about antimuscarinic medications before placement of an indwelling catheter is considered. Nevertheless, use of a catheter is often necessary for patients managed in a palliative care setting. Traditionally, indwelling catheters have been preferred, but external collection devices often provide a viable alternative to indwelling devices in men.

Functional UI is treated by minimizing barriers to toileting and the time required to prepare for urination.[6] Strategies designed to remove barriers to toileting are highly individualized and are best formulated with the use of a multidisciplinary team, combining nursing with medicine, as well as physical and occupational therapy as indicated.

Box 4.2 Pelvic Floor Muscle Contraction—the Knack

The knack describes a pelvic floor muscle contraction completed in response to physical exertion.

- The patient is taught to identify, contract, and relax the pelvic floor muscles, typically using some form of biofeedback.

- Biofeedback provides sensory, audible, or palpatory cues allowing the patient to identify the pelvic floor muscles and to differentiate contraction of these muscles from the abdominal, gluteal, or thigh muscles. Simple biofeedback maneuvers include assisting the patient to identify the pelvic floor muscles during a gentle vaginal or digital rectal examination, asking the patient to interrupt the urinary stream, or asking the patient to contract and relax while seated on a chair with a firm seat in order to maximize proprioception.

- After learning to identify, contract, and relax the pelvic floor muscles, the patient is taught to maximally contract (squeeze) these muscles when performing a maneuver associated with urine loss such as coughing, sneezing, walking, or bending over to don socks.

- This maneuver increases urethral closure and resistance to urinary incontinence (UI) and relieves or prevents stress UI. It is generally preferred in the palliative care setting because it provides some relief from stress UI within a comparatively brief period of time (usually within days to a week) compared with more formalized pelvic floor muscle training requiring 3 to 6 months.

Adapted from Miller JM, Ashton-Miller JA, Delancey JO. A pelvic muscle precontraction can reduce cough-related urine loss in selected women with mild SUI. *J Am Geriatr Soc.* 1998;46:870–874.

- Maximize mobility and access to the toilet by using assistive devices such as a walker or wheelchair, widening bathroom doors, adding support bars, and providing a bedside toilet or urinal.

- Reduce the time required for toileting by selected alterations in the patient's clothing, such as substituting tennis shoes with good traction for slippers or other footwear with slick soles and substituting Velcro- or elastic-banded clothing for articles with multiple buttons, zippers, or snaps.

- For patients with cognitive disorders, functional UI is usually managed by a prompted voiding program. The caregiver is taught to assist the patient to void on a fixed schedule, usually every 2 to 3 hours

Because extraurethral UI is caused by a fistulous tract and produces continuous urinary leakage, it must be managed initially by containment devices and preventive skin care. The type of containment device depends on the severity of the UI; an incontinent brief is frequently required. In some cases, the fistula may be closed by conservative (nonsurgical) means. An indwelling catheter is inserted, and the fistula is allowed to heal spontaneously. This intervention is most likely to work for a traumatic (postoperative) fistula. If the fistula is a result of an invasive tumor or radiation therapy, it is not as likely to heal

Table 4.3 Pharmacologic Management for Overactive Bladder and Urge Urinary Incontinence*

Antimuscarinic Drugs	Dosage	Nursing Considerations
Tolterodine ER (Detrol LA)	2–4 mg daily	May be administered at night to reduce dry mouth; administration with antacid or proton pump inhibitor may reduce bioavailability of drug; does not cross blood-brain barrier as readily as oxybutynin IR; the lower (2 mg) dose is recommended for patients with impaired hepatic function
Fesoterodine (Toviaz)	4–8 mg daily	Prodrug that is metabolized by ubiquitous esterases; metabolically active product is same as that for tolterodine; head-to-head trial demonstrated 8-mg dose superior to 4-mg dose
Oxybutynin IR (Ditropan IR)	5 mg twice daily to three times daily	Associated with higher incidence of moderate to severe dry mouth than extended release agents; readily crosses blood-brain barrier, potentially increasing the risk for central nervous side effects
Oxybutynin ER (Ditropan XL)	5–15 mg daily	Administered through osmotic releasing system; advise patient that skeleton of tablet will be passed in stool 24 to 48 hours after ingestion; incidence and severity of dry mouth less than IR formulation; may be administered at bedtime to reduce dry mouth
Oxybutynin TDS (Oxytrol)	3.9-mg patch twice weekly	Incidence of dry mouth not statistically different from placebo in pivotal trials; transdermal delivery system avoids first-pass effects of oral drug formulations, increasing bioavailability of drug; local skin irritation associated with use of patch not seen with oral agents
Oxybutynin transdermal gel (Gelnique)	Apply 1 package daily (equivalent to 10-mg daily dose)	Transdermal gel reduces likelihood of skin irritation associated with transdermal patch; incidence of dry mouth similar to oxybutynin patch
Solifenacin (VESIcare)	5–10 mg daily	Half-life of drug approximately 45–68 hours; may be administered at night to minimize dry mouth; use with caution in patients with impaired hepatic function
Darifenacin (Enablex)	7.5–15 mg daily	Drug has greater affinity for M3 muscarinic receptors; this receptor type is common in the bladder wall, bowel, and other peripheral organs, but absent in the central nervous system, reducing the potential for adverse central nervous system side effects; constipation rates reported in pivotal trial for this drug are higher than for other drugs, possibly associated with presence of M3 receptors in bowel wall

(continued)

Table 4.3 (Continued)

Antimuscarinic Drugs	Dosage	Nursing Considerations
Trospium ER (Sanctura XR)	60 mg daily	Drug is primarily excreted in urine rather than metabolized in liver, should be administered on empty stomach to maximize bioavailability; comparatively large size of trospium molecule (it is a quaternary amine) and lipophobic properties reduce likelihood drug will cross blood-brain barrier and produce central nervous system side effects
β_3-Agonist drugs:		
Mirabegron (Myrbetriq)	25–50 mg	New class of drug acts at β_3 receptors in bladder wall; avoids or reduces likelihood of specific adverse side effects of antimuscarinics such as dry mouth, flushing, or blurred vision; adverse side effects include hypertension

*These drugs are also used for managing painful bladder spasms because of their association with detrusor overactivity.

spontaneously. In such cases, cauterization and fibrin glue may be used to promote closure. Alternatively, a suspension containing tetracycline may be prepared and used as a sclerosing agent. The adjacent skin is prepared by applying a skin protectant (e.g., a petrolatum, dimethicone, or zinc oxide-based ointment) to protect it from the sclerosing agent. Approximately 5 to 10 mL of the tetracycline solution is injected into the fistula by a physician, and the lesion is monitored for signs of scarring and closure. If UI persists for 15 days or longer, the procedure may be repeated. For larger fistulas and those that fail to respond to conservative measures, surgical repair is undertaken if feasible.

Urinary Stasis and Retention

A precipitous drop or sudden cessation of urinary outflow is a serious urinary system complication that may indicate *oliguria* or *anuria* (failure of the kidneys to filter the blood and produce urine), *urinary stasis* (blockage of urine transport from the upper to lower urinary tracts), or *urinary retention* (failure of the bladder to evacuate itself of urine).

Urinary Stasis Due to Obstruction of the Upper Urinary Tract

Upper urinary tract stasis in the patient receiving palliative care is usually caused by obstruction of one or both ureters. The obstruction is typically attributable to a primary or metastatic tumor, and most arise from the pelvic region. In men, prostatic cancer is the most common cause, whereas pelvic (cervical, uterine, and ovarian) malignancies produce most ureteral obstructions in women. In addition to malignancies, retroperitoneal fibrosis secondary to inflammation or radiation may obstruct one or both ureters. Unless promptly relieved, bilateral ureteral obstruction leads to acute renal failure with uremia and elevated serum potassium, which can cause life-threatening arrhythmias. When a single ureter is obstructed, the bladder continues to fill with urine from the contralateral (unobstructed) kidney. In this case, urinary stasis produces symptoms of ureteral or renal colic. Left untreated, the affected kidney is prone to acute failure and infection, and it may produce systemic hypertension because of increased renin secretion.

Urinary Retention

Urinary retention is the inability to empty the urinary bladder despite micturition.

Acute urinary retention is an abrupt and complete inability to void. Patients are almost always aware of acute urinary retention because of the increasing suprapubic discomfort produced by bladder filling and distention and the associated anxiety.

Chronic urinary retention occurs when the patient is partly able to empty the bladder by voiding but a significant volume of urine remains behind. Although no absolute cutoff point for chronic urinary retention can be defined, most clinicians agree that a residual volume of 200 mL or more deserves further evaluation.

Assessment and Management of Upper Tract Obstruction and Urinary Retention

Accurate identification of the cause of a precipitous drop in urine output is essential because the management of upper urinary tract obstruction is different from that of urinary retention. Upper urinary tract obstruction is more likely to produce flank pain, usually localized to one or both flanks, although it may radiate to the abdomen and even to the labia or testes if the lower ureter is obstructed. Its intensity varies from moderate to intense. It typically is not relieved by changes in position, and the patient is often restless.

A focused physical examination assists the nurse to differentiate urinary retention from upper urinary tract obstruction. The patient with bilateral ureteral obstruction and acute renal failure may have systemic evidence of uremia, including nausea, vomiting, and hypertension. In some cases, obstruction may by complicated by pyelonephritis, causing a fever and chills. Physical assessment of the patient with upper urinary tract obstruction reveals a nondistended bladder, whereas the bladder is grossly distended and may extend above the umbilicus in the patient with acute urinary retention. Blood analysis reveals elevated serum creatinine, blood urea nitrogen, and potassium levels in the patient with bilateral ureteral obstruction, but these values are typically normal in the patient with urinary retention or unilateral ureteral obstruction. Ultrasonography of the kidneys and bladder reveals ureterohydronephrosis above the level of the obstruction or bladder distention in the patient with acute urinary retention.

Obstruction of the upper urinary tract is initially managed by reversal of fluid and electrolyte imbalances and prompt drainage.

- Urinary outflow can be reestablished by insertion of a ureteral stent (drainage tube extending from the renal pelvis to the bladder) through cystoscopy. A ureteral stent is preferred because it avoids the need for a percutaneous puncture and drainage bag. In the case of bilateral obstruction, a stent is placed in each ureter under endoscopic guidance; a single stent is placed if unilateral obstruction is diagnosed.

- If the ureter is significantly scarred because of radiation therapy or distorted because of a bulky tumor, placement of a ureteral stent may not be feasible, and a percutaneous nephrostomy tube may be required. The procedure may be done in an endoscopy suite or an interventional radiographic suite under local and systemic sedation or anesthesia. Unlike the ureteral stent that drains into the bladder, the nephrostomy tube is drained using a collection bag.

- Acute urinary retention is managed by prompt placement of an indwelling urinary catheter. The patient is closely monitored as the bladder is initially drained, because of the very small risk for brisk diuresis associated with transient hyperkalemia, hematuria, hypotension, and pallor. This risk may be further reduced by draining 500 mL, interrupted by a brief period during which the catheter is clamped (approximately 5 minutes), and followed by further drainage until the retained urine is evacuated. The catheter is left in place for up to 1 month, allowing the bladder to rest and recover from the overdistention typical of acute urinary retention.

- Chronic urinary retention may be managed by behavioral techniques, intermittent catheterization, or an indwelling catheter.[7] Behavioral methods are preferred because they are noninvasive and not associated with a risk for adverse side effects. Scheduled toileting with double voiding may be used in the patient with low urinary residual volumes (approximately 200 to 400 mL). The patient is taught to attempt voiding every 3 hours while awake and to double-void (urinate, wait for 3 to 5 minutes, and urinate again before leaving the bathroom). Higher urinary residual volumes and clinically relevant complications caused by urinary retention, including urinary tract infection or renal insufficiency, are usually managed by intermittent catheterization or an indwelling catheter.

Assessment and Management of Bothersome Lower Urinary Tract Symptoms and Bladder Spasm in Patients with Urinary Catheter or Stent

Irritative LUTS, including a heightened sense of urgency and urethral discomfort, are common in patients with a long-term indwelling catheter or ureteral stent. In certain cases, these irritative symptoms are accompanied by painful bladder spasms. Bladder spasms are characterized by intermittent episodes of excruciating, painful cramping localized to the suprapubic region. Painful bladder spasms may be the direct result of catheter occlusion by blood clots, sediment, or kinking; or they may be associated with a needlessly large catheter, an improperly inflated retention balloon, or hypersensitivity to the presence of the catheter or stent or to principal constituents. Other risk factors include pelvic radiation therapy, chemotherapeutic agents (particularly cyclophosphamide), intravesical tumors, urinary tract infections, and bladder or lower ureteral calculus.

Bladder spasms are managed by altering modifiable factors, administering anticholinergic medications, or employing more invasive therapies in highly selected cases.

- Changing the urethral catheter may relieve bladder spasms. An indwelling catheter is usually changed every 4 weeks or more often because of the risk for blockage and encrustation with precipitated salts, hardened urethral secretions, and bacteria.[8]

- A catheter with a smaller French size may be inserted if the catheter is larger than 16 French, unless the patient is experiencing a buildup of sediment causing catheter blockage.

- A catheter with a smaller retention balloon (5 mL) may be substituted for a catheter with a larger balloon (30 mL) to reduce irritation of the trigone and bladder neck.

- Use of a catheter that is constructed of hydrophilic polymers or latex-free silicone may relieve bladder spasms and diminish irritative LUTS because of their greater biocompatibility compared with Teflon-coated catheters.

- In certain cases, such as when the urethral catheter produces significant urethritis with purulent discharge from the urethra, a suprapubic indwelling catheter may be substituted for the urethral catheter. A suprapubic catheter also may be placed in patients who have a urethra that is technically difficult to catheterize or in those in whom the catheter tends to encrust despite adequate fluid intake. Once established, these catheters are changed monthly, usually in the outpatient, home care, or hospice setting.

If conservative measures or catheter modifications fail to relieve bladder spasms, an anticholinergic medication may be administered. These medications work by inhibiting the overactive contractions that lead to painful bladder spasms.

Hematuria

Hematuria is defined as the presence of blood in the urine. It results from a variety of renal, urologic, and systemic processes. In the palliative care setting, hematuria may be associated with a variety of disorders, including pelvic irradiation or chemotherapy, or may result from a major coagulation disorder or a newly diagnosed or recurring malignancy.

Hematuria is divided into two subtypes according to its clinical manifestations. Microscopic hematuria is characterized by hemoglobin or myoglobin on dipstick analysis and more than 3 to 5 red blood cells (RBCs) per high-power field (hpf) under microscopic urinalysis, but the presence of blood remains invisible to the unaided eye. Macroscopic (gross) hematuria is also characterized by dipstick and microscopic evidence of RBCs in the urine, as well as a bright red or brownish discoloration that is apparent to the unaided eye.

In the context of palliative care, hematuria can also be subdivided into three categories depending on its severity.

- Mild hematuria is microscopic or gross blood in the urine that does not produce obstructing clots or cause a clinically relevant decline in hematocrit or hemoglobin.

- Moderate and severe hematuria are associated with more prolonged and high-volume blood losses; hematuria is classified as moderate if less than

6 units of blood are required to replace blood lost within the urine and as severe if 6 units or more are required. Both moderate and severe hematuria may produce obstructing clots that lead to acute urinary retention or obstruction of the upper urinary tract.

Assessment

A careful, detailed history is needed to identify the source of the bleeding and to initiate an appropriate treatment plan. The patient should be asked whether the hematuria represents a new, persistent, or recurrent problem. A review of prior urinalyses also may provide clues to the onset and history of microscopic hematuria in particular. The patient is queried about the relation of grossly visible hematuria to the urinary stream. Bleeding limited to initiation of the stream is often associated with a urethral source, bleeding during the entire act of voiding usually indicates a source in the bladder or upper urinary tract, and bleeding near the termination of the stream often indicates a source within the prostate or male reproductive system.

The patient with gross hematuria should also be asked about the color of the urine: a bright red hue indicates fresh blood, whereas a darker hue (often described as brownish, rust, or "Coke" colored) indicates older blood. Some patients with severe hematuria report the passage of blood clots. Clots that are particularly long and thin, resembling a shoestring or fishhook, suggest an upper urinary tract source; larger and bulkier clots suggest a lower urinary tract source.

The patient is asked about any pain related to the hematuria; this questioning should include the site and character of the pain and any radiation of pain to the flank, lower abdomen, or groin. Flank pain usually indicates upper urinary tract problems, abdominal pain radiating to the groin usually indicates lower ureteral obstruction and bleeding, and suprapubic pain suggests obstruction or infection causing hematuria.

In addition to questions about the hematuria, the nurse should ask about specific risk factors, including a history of urinary tract infections; systemic symptoms suggesting infection or renal insufficiency, including fever, weight loss, rash, and recent systemic infection; any history of primary or metastatic tumors of the genitourinary system; and chemotherapy or radiation therapy of the pelvic or lower abdominal region. A focused review of medications includes all chemotherapeutic agents used currently or in the past and any current or recent administration of anticoagulant medications, including warfarin, heparin, aspirin, nonsteroidal anti-inflammatory drugs, and other anticoagulant agents.

Physical Examination

Physical examination also provides valuable clues to the source of hematuria. When completing this assessment, the nurse should particularly note any abdominal masses or tenderness, skin rashes, bruising, purpura (suggesting vasculitis, bleeding, or coagulation disorders), or telangiectasia (suggesting von Hippel-Lindau disease). Blood pressure should be assessed because a new onset or rapid exacerbation of hypertension may suggest a renal source for hematuria. The lower abdomen is examined for signs of bladder distention, and a rectal assessment is completed to evaluate apparent prostatic or rectal masses or induration.

Laboratory Testing and Imaging

A dipstick and microscopic urinalysis is usually combined with microscopic examination when evaluating hematuria. This provides a semiquantitative assessment of the severity of hematuria (RBCs/hpf), and it excludes pseudohematuria (reddish urine caused by something other than RBCs, such as ingestion of certain drugs, vegetable dyes, or pigments).

Urinalysis provides further clues to the likely source of the bleeding. Dysmorphic RBCs, cellular casts, renal tubular cells, and proteinuria indicate upper urinary tract bleeding. In contrast, hematuria from the lower urinary tract is usually associated with normal RBC morphology.

Ultrasonography is almost always indicated in the evaluation of hematuria in the patient receiving palliative care. It is used to identify the size and location of cystic or solid masses that may act as the source of hematuria and to assess for obstruction, most stones, larger blood clots, and bladder-filling defects. A computed tomography intravenous pyelogram or a magnetic resonance imaging urogram also may be used to image the upper and lower urinary tracts, but clinical use is limited by the risk for contrast allergy or nephropathy. Cystoscopy is performed if a bladder lesion is suspected, and ureteroscopy with retrograde pyelography may be completed if an upper urinary tract source of bleeding is suspected.

Management

The management of hematuria is guided by its severity and its source or cause. Table 4.4 summarizes treatment options for moderate to severe hematuria and their route, administration, and principal nursing considerations.[9,10]

Table 4.4 Treatment Options for Hemorrhagic Cystitis		
Agent	**Action, Route of Administration, and Dosage**	**Problems and Contraindications**
ε-Aminocaproic acid	Acts as an inhibitor of fibrinolysis by inhibiting plasminogen activation substances 5-g loading dose orally or parenterally, followed by 1-1.25 g hourly to maximum of 30 g in 24 hr Maximum response in 8-12 hr	Potential thromboembolic complications Increased risk for clot retention Contraindicated in patients with upper urinary tract bleeding or vesicoureteral reflux Decreased blood pressure
Silver nitrate	Chemical cautery Intravesical instillation: 0.5% to 1.0% solution in sterile water instilled for 10–20 min followed by no irrigation; multiple instillations may be required Reported as 68% effective	Case report of renal failure in patient who precipitated silver salts in renal collecting system, causing functional obstruction

(continued)

Table 4.4 (Continued)

Agent	Action, Route of Administration, and Dosage	Problems and Contraindications
Alum (may use ammonium or potassium salt of aluminum)	Chemical cautery Continuous bladder irrigation: 1% solution in sterile water, pH = 4.5 (salt precipitates at pH of 7) Requires average of 21 hr of treatment	Thought to not be absorbed by bladder mucosa; however, case reports of aluminum toxicity in renal failure patients
Formalin (aqueous solution of formaldehyde)	Cross-links proteins; exists as monohydrate methylene glycol and as a mixture of polymeric hydrates and polyoxyethylene glycols; rapidly "fixes" the bladder mucosa Available as 37%–40%, aqueous formaldehyde (=100% formalin) diluted in sterile water to desired concentration (1% formalin = 0.37% formaldehyde) Instillation: 50 mL for 4-10 min or endoscopic placement of 5% formalin-soaked pledgets placed onto bleeding site for 15 min and then removed	Painful, requires anesthesia Vesicoureteral reflux (relative contraindication): patients placed in Trendelenburg position with low-grade reflux or ureteral occlusive balloons used with high-grade reflux Extravasation causes fibrosis, papillary necrosis, fistula, peritonitis
Intravesical prostaglandins	Prostaglandin E_1 (PGE_1) PGE_2, and $PGF_{2\alpha}$ may be used to treat cyclophosphamide-induced hematuria Prostaglandins are postulated to act by promoting platelet aggregation, vasoconstriction through contraction of smooth muscles of arterioles in mucosa and submucosa, and a cytoprotective action influencing glycosaminoglycan function of the urothelium Prostaglandins are introduced following introduction of a three-way indwelling catheter and evacuation of clots; PGE_1, PGE_2, and $PGF_{2\alpha}$ are introduced in a diluted aqueous solution and retained in the bladder for approximately 1 hour Dosing varies according to the individual formulations Multiple treatments are required (median 6–7 days reported in several case series) Gross hematuria resolves in approximately 50% of cases	Bladder spasms commonly occur; nevertheless are associated with less systemic toxicity than formalin Treatment may be administered at the bedside

Adapted from Ghahstani SM, Shakhssalim N. Palliative treatment of intractable hematuria in context of advanced bladder cancer. *Urology.* 2009;6(3):149–156; and Groninger H, Phillips JM. Gross hematuria: assessment and management at end of life. *J Hospice Palliat Nurs.* 2012;14(3):184–188.

Conclusion

Patients receiving palliative care frequently experience urinary system disorders. A malignancy or systemic disease may affect voiding function and produce UI, urinary retention, or upper urinary tract obstruction. In addition, upper acute renal insufficiency or renal failure may occur if the upper urinary tract becomes obstructed. These disorders may be directly attributable to a malignancy or systemic disease, or they may be caused by a specific treatment such as radiation, chemotherapy, or a related medication. Nursing management of patients with urinary system disorders is affected by the nature of the urologic condition, the patient's general condition, and the nearness to death.

References

1. Abrams P, Cardozo L, Fall M, et al. The standardization of terminology of lower urinary tract function: report for the standardization sub-committee of the International Continence Society. *Neurourol Urodyn.* 2002;*21*:167–178.

2. Wilson M. Causes and management of indwelling urinary catheter-related pain. *Br J Nurs.* 2008;*17*:232–239.

3. Gray M, Beeckman D, Bliss DZ, et al. Incontinence-associated dermatitis: a comprehensive review and update. *J Wound Ostomy Continence Nurs.* 2012; *39*(1)61–74.

4. Miller JM, Ashton-Miller JA, Delancey JO. A pelvic muscle precontraction can reduce cough-related urine loss in selected women with mild SUI. *J Am Geriatr Soc.* 1998;*46*:870–874.

5. MacDiarmid SA. How to choose the initial drug treatment for overactive bladder. *Curr Urol Rep.* 2007;*8*:364–369.

6. Fink HA, Taylor BC, Tacklind, JW, et al. Treatment interventions in nursing home residents with urinary incontinence: a systematic review of randomized trials. *Mayo Clin Proc.* 2008;*83*(12):1332–1343.

7. Newman DK. The indwelling urinary catheter: principles for best practice. *J Wound Ostomy Continence Nurs.* 2007;*34*:655–661.

8. Parker D, Callan L, Harwood J, et al. Nursing interventions to reduce the risk of catheter-associated urinary tract infection. Part 1: catheter selection. *J Wound Ostomy Continence Nurs.* 2009;*36*:23–34.

9. Ghahstani SM, Shakhssalim N. Palliative treatment of intractable hematuria in context of advanced bladder cancer. *Urology.* 2009;*6*(3):149–156.

10. Groninger H. Phillips JM. Gross hematuria: assessment and management at end of life. *J Hospice Palliat Nurs.* 2012;*14*(3):184–188.

Chapter 5

Lymphedema Management

Mei R. Fu

Introduction

Lymphedema, or abnormal swelling, is seen regularly in palliative and acute care settings. Lymphedema is often overlooked or neglected despite its capacity to cause pain, immobility, infection, skin problems, and psychosocial distress.[1] Because nurses have access to large, diverse patient populations, they constitute an ideal resource for providing and improving quality care for patients suffering from lymphedema.

Definitions

Lymphedema is a chronic syndrome of abnormal swelling and multiple symptoms, resulting from abnormal accumulation of protein-rich lymph fluid in the interstitial tissue spaces due to an imbalance between lymph fluid production and transport.[2] *Edema*, a symptom, refers to excessive accumulation of fluid within interstitial tissues and is one of the manifestations of lymphedema.[2] Long-term, neglected edema, such as lower extremity venous insufficiency, can develop into chronic lymphedema. Discerning the difference between edema and lymphedema allows appropriate treatment. Lymphedema and edema are contrasted in Table 5.1,[1-3] which provides definitions, signs and symptoms, and basic pathophysiology.

Prevalence and Risk Factors

Primary lymphedema, a genetic disorder, is attributed to embryonic developmental abnormalities, which may be sporadic or part of a syndrome caused by either chromosomal abnormalities (e.g., Turner's syndrome) or inherited single-gene defects. Primary lymphedema occurs in about one in 6,000 individuals and is more common in women than men.

Secondary (acquired) lymphedema results from obstruction or obliteration of lymph nodes or lymphatic vessels.[2] Cancer, trauma, surgery, severe infections, cardiac disease, poor venous function, immobility, and paralyzing diseases are major causes of secondary lymphedema.[2,4] In developing countries, lymphatic filariasis, a parasitic infection transmitted by mosquitoes, is the predominant worldwide cause of secondary lymphedema. Mosquitoes

Table 5.1 Definitions, Signs, and Symptoms of Edema Versus Lymphedema

	Edema	Lymphedema
Disorder	A symptom of various disorders	A chronic, currently incurable edema
Definition	Swelling caused by the excessive fluid in interstitial tissues—due to imbalance between capillary filtration and lymph drainage over time	Swelling (edema) caused by accumulation of lymph fluid within interstitial tissues as a result of lymphatic drainage failure, increased production of lymph fluid over time, or both
Signs and symptoms	Swelling, decreased skin mobility	Swelling, decreased skin mobility
	Tightness, tingling, or bursting	Tightness, heaviness, firmness, tingling, feeling of fullness, or bursting sensations
	Decreased strength and mobility	Decreased strength and mobility
	Discomfort (aching to severe pain)	Discomfort (aching, soreness to severe pain)
	Possible skin color change	Progressive skin changes (color, texture, tone, temperature), integrity such as blisters, weeping (lymphorrhea), hyperkeratosis, warts, papillomatosis, and elephantiasis
	Pitting scale is often used:	*Pitting scale is NOT used*
	1+ Edema barely detectable	
	2+ Slight indentation with depression	
	3+ Deep indentation for 5–30 sec with pressure	
	4+ Area 1.5–2 times greater than normal	
Pathophysiology	Capillary filtration rate exceeds fluid transport capacity	Inadequate lymph transport capacity
		Primary—Inadequately developed lymphatic pathways
	Example: Heart failure, fluid overload, and venous thrombosis are common causes of increased capillary pressure, leading to an increased capillary filtration rate that causes edema	*Secondary*—Damage outside lymphatic pathways (obstruction/obliteration)
		Initial sequelae of transport failure:
		Lymphatic stasis →

(continued)

Table 5.1 (Continued)

Edema	Lymphedema
	Increased tissue fluid →
Note:	Accumulated protein and cellular metabolites →
Timely treatment of the underlying cause or causes usually reduces edema	Further increased tissue water and pressure
	Potential long-term sequelae:
Prolonged, untreated edema can transition to lymphedema	Macrophages seek to decrease inflammation
	Increased fibroblasts and keratinocytes cause chronic inflammation
	Gradual increase in adipose tissue
	Lymphorrhea (leakage of lymph through skin)
	Gradual skin and tissue thickening and hardening progressing to hyperkeratosis, papillomatosis, and other problems
	Ever-increasing risk for infection and other complications

Adapted from references 1, 2, and 3.

transmit filariasis nematodes, which embed in human lymphatics to cause progressive lymphatic damage.

In developed countries, cancer treatment is the main cause of lymphedema. Prevalence of cancer-related lymphedema has been reported in patients treated for breast cancer (5% to 60%), melanoma (16%), gynecologic cancer (20%), genitourinary cancer (10%), and head or neck cancer (4%).[4] Risk factors related to cancer treatment include extent of surgery, extent of lymph node resection, and radiation therapy.[4–6]

Inflammation, infection, and higher body mass index are the main predictors of lymphedema besides cancer treatment-related risk.[5,6] Breast cancer survivors who underwent surgery and dissection of lymph nodes and vessels are known to have a compromised lymphatic system, which makes them more vulnerable to infection and ineffective lymphatic drainage. Nevertheless, these risk factors only partially explain who develops lymphedema, and lymphedema can and does occur in people lacking these risk factors.

Impact

Often, the most visible manifestation of lymphedema is persistent swelling.[1-3] Yet, lymphedema is more than swelling alone. Lymphedema exerts extensive impact on an individual's quality of life, including physical discomfort, functional disabilities, impaired occupational roles, poor self-image, decreased self-esteem, interrupted interpersonal relationships, financial burden, and lifestyle changes. [1,7,8] Physically, lymphedema leads to distressing symptoms such as swelling, firmness, tightness, heaviness, pain, fatigue, numbness, and impaired limb mobility. [2,7] Lymphedema also predisposes individuals to fibrosis, cellulitis, infections, lymphadenitis, or septicemia. Prolonged fluid stasis can lead to severe skin and tissue symptoms, sometimes referred to as *elephantiasis*. Symptoms include hyperkeratosis (hard, reptile-like skin), warts, and papillomas (engorged and raised lymph vessels on the skin surface). Chronic lymphedema, over a number of years, has also been associated with the development of the rare, usually fatal cancer, lymphangiosarcoma. Functionally, lymphedema makes it difficult for individuals to accomplish tasks and impairs their abilities to fulfill work that involves heavy lifting, gripping, holding, fine motor dexterity, and repetitive movement of the affected limb. [7] Psychologically, individuals feel stigmatized and a loss of sexual attractiveness because of obvious disfigurement, which often elicits emotional distress, social anxiety, depression, and disruption of interpersonal relationships. [1] Financially, routine checkups for lymphedema management, long-term physical therapy, management equipment (compression garments, bandages, special lotions), and repeated cellulitis, infections, and lymphangitis create financial and economic burdens not only for survivors but also to the healthcare system. [8] Breast cancer survivors with lymphedema have significantly higher health care costs than those without, they spend more days annually either hospitalized or visiting physicians' offices; and they have more days absent from work, which could adversely affect employment. [8]

Assessment and Diagnosis

Diagnosing lymphedema remains a clinical challenge. Several factors contribute to the challenge: lack of universally recognized diagnostic criteria; failure to precisely evaluate symptoms; coexisting conditions; and lack of awareness of lymphedema among health care professionals. To ensure accurate diagnosis, it is important to conduct a careful review of the patient's health history to exclude other medical conditions that may cause similar symptoms, such as recurrent cancer, deep vein thrombosis, chronic venous insufficiency, diabetes, hypertension, and cardiac and renal disease. These alternative diagnoses should be ruled out before establishing a diagnosis of lymphedema and referring the patient for lymphedema therapy. Box 5.1 describes the sequential components of a lymphedema assessment.

Assessment of Symptoms

Symptom assessment is essential because very often observable swelling and measurable volume changes are absent during the initial development of lymphedema. [3] Table 5.2 presents an example of a symptom checklist for breast cancer–related lymphedema. [3] These symptoms may be the earliest

Box 5.1 Sequential Components of Lymphedema Assessment

Rule out or address immediate complications (i.e., infection, thrombosis, severe pain, new or recurrent cancer, significant nonrelated disorders)

History and physical examination

Routine physical assessments: vital signs, blood pressure, height and weight, body mass index

Past and current health status, including medications and allergies (especially antibiotic allergies and history of infection, trauma, or surgery in affected area)

Current activities of daily living (job, home responsibilities, leisure activities, sleep position, activities that aggravate lymphedema)

Current psychological health, support people, view of lymphedema and health

History of lymphedema etiology, presentation, duration, and progression

Patient knowledge of and response to lymphedema, interest in assistance and goals

Third-party payer status

Quantification of lymphedema status (lymphedema signs and symptoms, volume, pain and other neurologic symptoms, tissue status, range of motion of nearby joints, site-specific and overall patient function)

indicator of increasing interstitial pressure changes associated with lymphedema.[3] As the fluid increases, the limb may become visibly swollen with an observable increase in limb size. Because lymphedema symptoms elicit tremendous distress and impair quality of life, they should warrant institution of early interventions.[7] Resolution of symptoms should be one of the major patient-centered clinical outcomes for evaluating the effectiveness of lymphedema treatment.

Questionable clinical symptoms or etiology may require further evaluation. Lymphoscintigraphy (isotope lymphography) can ensure definite lymphedema diagnosis.[3] Assessment for infection, thrombosis, or cancer metastasis is required at every patient contact. Although later signs of infection or thrombosis are well known, awareness and careful assessment allow early diagnosis and treatment. Lymphedema progression or treatment resistance may be the earliest sign of complication or may represent a lack of response to current treatment. Changes in pain or comfort, skin (color, temperature, condition), or mobility and range of motion are other possible early signs of major complications. Most infections develop subcutaneously, beneath intact skin. Cultures are not recommended because they rarely document a bacterial source and can further increase the risk for infection. Suspected thrombosis or new or recurring cancer requires appropriate diagnostic evaluation (e.g., Doppler ultrasonography, magnetic resonance imaging, positron emission tomography, computed tomographic scanning). Venous ultrasonography is reported to be safer than venography for evaluation of suspected thrombosis in a limb with, or at high risk for, lymphedema.

Table 5.2 Example of Symptom Checklist: Breast Cancer and Lymphedema Symptom Experience Index

The following questions are about symptoms in your affected arm, hand, breast, axilla (under arm), or chest today or in the past three months.

	How Severe?				
Have you had ___?	**No** 0	**A little** 1	**Somewhat** 2	**Quite a bit** 3	**Very Severe** 4
1. Limited shoulder movement					
2. Limited elbow movement					
3. Limited wrist movement					
4. Limited fingers movement					
5. Limited arm movement					
6. Hand or arm swelling					
7. Breast swelling					
8. Chest wall swelling					
9. Firmness					
10. Tightness					
11. Heaviness					
12. Toughness or thickness of skin					
13. Stiffness					
14. Tenderness					
15. Hotness/increased temperature					
16. Redness					
17. Blistering					
18. Pain/aching/ soreness					
19. Numbness					
20. Burning					
21. Stabbing					
22. Tingling (pins and needles)					
23. Arm or hand fatigue					
24. Arm or hand weakness					

Quantification of Lymphedema

A variety of measurement approaches make quantification of lymphedema a problem. Methods of measuring limb volume or circumference include sequential circumference limb measurement, water displacement, and infrared perometry.[9] The most clinically useful tool is measuring the limb, although this has limited utility when trying to quantify lymphedema that occurs in the face, neck, shoulder, breast, abdomen, thoracic regions, or genital areas.

Sequential Circumferential Arm Measurements

Measuring limb volume and circumference is the most widely used diagnostic method. A flexible nonstretch tape measure for circumferences is usually used to assure consistent tension over soft tissue, muscle, and bony prominences.[9] Measurements are done on both affected and nonaffected limbs at the hand proximal to the metacarpals, wrist, and then every 4 cm from the wrist to axilla. The most common criterion for diagnosis has been a finding of at least a 2-cm or 200-mL difference in limb volume compared with the nonaffected limb or a 10% volume difference in the affected limb.[9]

Lymphedema Risk Reduction

Patient education focusing on risk reduction strategies holds great promise for reducing the risk for lymphedema. Breast cancer survivors who received lymphedema information reported significantly fewer symptoms and more practice of risk reduction behaviors than those who did not.

- Maintain an ideal body weight because excess body weight is associated with decreased lymphatic function.[10]
- Infection prevention is vital for lymphedema risk reduction; risk increases with breaches in skin integrity.[10]
    - Limit drawing of blood.
    - Request an experienced phlebotomist and emphasize the patient's increased infection risk.
    - Weigh the risks and benefits of central venous catheter use with venipuncture.
    - Diabetes potentially increases breast cancer patients' lymphedema risk when the affected limb is used for continual blood sticks or insulin injections.
    - Patients with bilateral limb risk, especially of the upper extremities, face lifelong decisions regarding adherence to precautions.
- Encourage use of a compression sleeve at the earliest sign of edema.
- Cancer survivors should be encouraged to carry out all postoperative exercises, resume normal precancer activities, and be as fit as possible, while regularly monitoring their high-risk or affected limb.[11] Individuals should be instructed to perform physical exercise according to the general exercise guidelines: (1) initiate at lower intensity exercise; then graduate to increase exercise intensity; (2) exercise to the extent that the affected body part is not fatigued; (3) modify physical exercise to reduce the risk for trauma and injury; and (4) use a compression garment during exercise.

Long-Term Management

Edema usually subsides with proper treatment, whereas lymphedema requires long-term management.[12] Long-term management focuses on daily activities and strategies undertaken to decrease the swelling, relieve symptom distress, and prevent acute exacerbations and infections (Box 5.2).[12]

Long-term management necessitates a multidisciplinary approach. At each patient visit, nurses should assess for signs of infection, limb confirmation, and degree of swelling. Additional inquiries need to be made as to any other symptoms patients may be experiencing because of the lymphedema. Nurses should assess self-care behaviors and encourage patients with lymphedema to wear their compression sleeves as prescribed, which includes during activities such as flying and exercise.[12] Antibiotics may be prescribed for infections. Patients with new-onset or worsening lymphedema should be referred to certified lymphedema therapists for volume reduction treatment. Certified lymphedema therapists should provide treatment for the swollen limb and individualized patient education about self-care practices (including recommended exercise and exercise progression based on individual lymphedema risk factors and level of fitness).

Infection Prevention and Treatment

Infection is the most common lymphedema complication. Lymphatic stasis, decreased local immune response, tissue congestion, and accumulated proteins and other debris foster infection. Traditional signs and symptoms (fever, malaise, lethargy, and nausea) are often present. Prompt oral or intravenous antibiotic therapy is indicated. Because streptococci and staphylococci are frequent precipitators, antibiotics must cover normal skin flora, as well as gram-positive cocci, and have good skin penetration.[13] Early detection and treatment can help prevent the need for intravenous therapy and hospitalization.[13] Intravenous antibiotic therapy is recommended for systemic signs of infection or insufficient response to oral antibiotics.

Nursing activities include assisting patients in obtaining prompt antibiotic therapy, monitoring and reporting signs and symptoms, and providing instruction regarding high fluid intake, rest, elevation of the infected limb, and

---

Box 5.2 Components of Long-Term Lymphedema Management

History, physical examination, and ongoing assessment and support
Individualized and holistic care coordination
Multi-disciplined referrals
Comprehensive initial and ongoing patient instruction
Ongoing psychosocial support
Promotion of ongoing optimal self-care management
Facilitation of appropriate evidence-based, individualized treatment
Patient and practice outcome measurement
Access and long-term follow-up and management
Communication and collaboration with related health care providers

avoidance of strenuous activity. Garment-type compression is encouraged as soon as tolerable during infection. Infection prophylaxis has been highly effective for patients who experience repeated serious infections or inflammatory episodes. Effective edema reduction and control may also help prevent lymphedema infection.

The feet, which are especially susceptible to fungal infections in lower extremity lymphedema, can exhibit peeling, scaly skin, and toenail changes. Antifungal powders are recommended prophylactically. Antifungal creams should be used at the first sign of fungus. Diabetic-like skin care and use of cotton socks and well-fitted, breathable (leather or canvas), sturdy shoes are beneficial.[13]

Self-Care

Optimal patient self-care typically includes adherence to risk reduction behaviors, use of compression, weight management, fitness and lymphedema exercises, optimal nutrition and hydration, healthy lifestyle practices, and seeking assistance for lymphedema-related problems.[12] Patient empowerment for optimal self-care is a great impetus to long-term management success.

Elevation
Elevation of the affected limb above the level of the heart is often recommended to reduce swelling. Elevation promotes the drainage of lymph fluid by maximizing venous drainage and by decreasing capillary pressure and lymph production. Elevation is considered the main treatment for early-stage lymphedema of an upper limb. Anecdotal evidence suggests that limb elevation when the patient is sitting or in bed may be a useful adjunct to active treatment, but should not be allowed to impede function or activity. Patients should be encouraged not to sleep in a chair but to go to bed at night to avoid the development of "arm chair" legs or exacerbation of lower limb lymphedema. Patient avoidance of limb dependency is also an appropriate risk reduction strategy and ameliorates the symptoms of lymphedema.

Exercise
Exercise or body movement is an integral part of lymphedema management and risk reduction. Exercise improves muscular strength, cardiovascular function, psychological well-being, and functional capacity.[11] Gentle resistance exercise stimulates muscle pumps and increases lymph flow; aerobic exercise increases intra-abdominal pressure, which facilitates pumping of the thoracic duct.[11] A tailored exercise or body movement program that combines flexibility, resistance, and aerobic exercise may be beneficial in reducing the risk for, and controlling, lymphedema. General exercise guidelines include the following:

- Start with low- to moderate-intensity exercise.
- Walking, swimming, cycling, and low-impact aerobics are recommended.
- Flexibility exercises should be performed to maintain range of movement.
- Appropriate warming-up and cooling-down phases should be implemented as part of exercise to avoid exacerbation of swelling.
- Heavy lifting and repetitive motion should be avoided.
- Compression garments should be worn during exercise.

Skin Care

Skin care is important for lymphedema risk reduction and management, which optimizes the condition of the skin and prevents infection. Diligent care is especially important for patients with lower extremity, genital, breast, head, neck, or late-stage lymphedema, additional skin alterations, or unrelated debilitating conditions. Lymphedema can cause skin dryness and irritation, which is increased with long-term use of compression products. Bland, nonscented products are recommended for daily cleansing and moisturizing. Low-pH moisturizers, which discourage infection, are recommended for advanced lymphedema because skin and tissue changes increase infection risk. Water-based moisturizers, which are absorbed more readily, are less likely to damage compression products but are not suitable for all patients. Cotton clothing allows ventilation and is absorbent.

Advanced lymphedema can cause several skin complications, including lymphorrhea, lymphoceles, papillomas, and hyperkeratosis. Lymphorrhea is leakage of lymph fluid through the skin that occurs when skin cannot accommodate accumulated fluid. Nonadherent dressings, good skin care, and compression are used to alleviate leakage. Compression and good skin care also reduce the occurrence of lymphoceles, papillomas, and hyperkeratosis; these complications reflect skin adaptation to excess subcutaneous lymph.

Bandages

Multi-layer lymphedema bandaging (MLLB) provides external compression. For some patients, MLLB may be used as part of long-term or palliative management. MLLB uses inelastic or low-stretch bandages to produce a massaging effect and stimulate lymph flow. MLLB is especially important for patients with severe lymphedema, such as lymphedema with morbid obesity or neglected primary lymphedema. Foam or other padding is often used under bandages to improve edema reduction and foster limb uniformity. The time, effort, and dexterity required for bandaging can become burdensome or impossible for some patients, necessitating the use of an alternative compression method.[14]

MLLB should be avoided for the following conditions:

- Severe arterial insufficiency
- Uncontrolled heart failure
- Severe peripheral neuropathy[14]

Some components of the MLLB system can be washed and dried according to the manufacturer's instructions and reused. Over time, inelastic bandages progressively lose their extensibility, which will increase their stiffness. Heavily soiled, cohesive, and adhesive bandages should be discarded after use.[14]

Compression Garments

Compression garments are recommended for patients with lymphedema of the extremities.[15] Compression garments can be used as initial management in patients who have mild upper or lower limb lymphedema (International Society of Lymphology stage I) with minor pitting, no significant tissue changes, no or minimal shape distortion, or palliative needs. Physiologic effects of compression include edema control or reduction, decreased accumulated protein, decreased arteriole outflow into the interstitium, improved muscle pump effect with movement and exercise of the affected area, and protection of skin. Patients should be reviewed 4 to 6 weeks after initial fitting, and then at each garment renewal approximately every 3 to 6 months.[14]

Garment use requires frequent laundering of products (daily to every other day), daily skin care and complication monitoring, and two replacements every 6 months. Various helpful products are available to assist patients in applying garments—an especially important task for elderly and disabled patients. Hand arthritis or neuropathy can hinder tolerance of garments. Garment removal is required if compression causes pain, neurologic symptoms, or color or temperature changes. Readjustment and movement may remedy the problem; often, product replacement is required. Because a variety of products exist, staff and patient persistence is likely to result in good patient tolerance. Rubber gloves (dishwashing gloves) facilitate application of garments and extend their longevity. Timely garment replacement (usually every 6 months) is essential for good edema control.[14]

Decongestive Lymphatic Therapy and Lymph Drainage Massage

Decongestive lymphatic therapy includes manual lymph drainage, multi-layer, short-stretch compression bandaging, gentle remedial upper limb exercise, meticulous skin care, education in lymphedema self-management, and elastic compression garments, and has become the standard of care for treating lymphedema.[14] Patients generally receive 2-hour treatments 5 days a week for 3 to 8 weeks, requiring them to make a commitment to continue performing the exercise and skin care, as well as wearing the compression garments. Compliance with the prescribed treatment is difficult because even the most customized garments or sleeves sometimes are uncomfortable, unsightly, and laborious to put on.[14] A constellation of complex factors (e.g., physical, financial, aesthetic, time) can influence survivors' compliance with treatment. For treatment to be maximally effective, lymphedema needs to be treated by therapists with special training and experience in this field.

Pneumatic (Mechanical) Pumps

Mechanical pumps use electricity to inflate a single-chamber or multi-chamber sleeve and produce external limb compression. A decreased tissue capillary filtration rate (documented by lymphoscintigraphy) produces tissue fluid reduction and, consequently, limb volume decrease.[15] Lymph formation decreases, but lymph transport, which would address lymphedema pathophysiology, is not affected. Pneumatic pumps can reduce swelling, but concern exists regarding the way in which swelling is decreased as well as the rapid displacement of fluid elsewhere in the body. In addition, the use of pumps does not eliminate the need for compression garments and may not provide more benefit than garments alone.[15] Using pumps may cause complications, including lymphatic congestion and injury proximal to the pump sleeve, increased swelling adjacent to the pump cuff in up to 18% of patients, lack of benefit in all but stage I (reversible) lymphedema, and development of genital

> **Box 5.3 Nursing Interventions for Lymphedema Secondary to Cancer of the Head and Neck**
>
> - Help patients to make an informed decision in a supportive environment.
> - Instruction and support in establishment of a lifelong daily self-care regimen, including range-of-motion exercises, skin assessment, and application of moisturizers; early, skilled patient complication assistance; and use of safe external compression. A written self-care program may foster patient self-care adherence.
> - Monitor external neck compression. External neck compression must provide sufficient pressure to stimulate lymphatic function without causing skin irritation/injury or impairment of breathing, eating, or swallowing.
> - Encourage daily self-care using manual lymph drainage to further improve edema control.
> - Document patient outcomes, including interval neck circumferences, skin integrity, pain level, and neck range of motion.

lymphedema in up to 43% of patients with cancer-related lower extremity lymphedema.[15] After more than 50 years of pump use in lymphedema care and long-established Medicare reimbursement, no guidelines exist, significant complications are reported, and research has not clarified benefit.

Unusual Lymphedemas

Palliative care may require the management of unusual and challenging lymphedema sites, such as breast, head, neck, trunk, or genitals. Manual drainage, skin-softening techniques, foam chip pads, and external compression (if possible) are recommended. External compression may be achieved with collars, vests, custom pants or tights, scrotal supports, or spandex-type exercise apparel. The assistance of occupational or physical therapists and a seamstress may be helpful.

Lymphedema secondary to head and neck cancer commonly presents following surgery and radiotherapy. Lymphedema is frequently found below the chin in the anterior neck. Difficult in swallowing and breathing are the major symptom distress from neck lymphedema. Mild swelling often progresses fairly rapidly to firm, nonpitting swelling; this may often not be recognized or treated as lymphedema. Box 5.3 presents detailed information about nursing interventions for neck lymphedema from head and neck cancer.[13]

Conclusion

Edema is a symptom usually relieved by addressing the causative factor. Lymphedema is a chronic disorder that requires long-term management. Although external compression is essential to effective lymphedema management, third-party payer reimbursement is inadequate and frustrating, patients are frequently fitted with products they cannot tolerate, and many patients have not been adequately prepared for compression products and therefore discontinue use when their product does not cure the lymphedema. Nevertheless, over the last two decades, progress has been achieved in both lymphedema awareness and scientific research and nurses have played a key role in advancing this field.

References

1. Fu MR, Ridner SH, Hu SH, et al. Psychosocial impact of lymphedema: a systematic review of literature from 2004 to 2011. *Psycho-Oncol*. 2013;*22*(7):1466–1484.

2. Chachaj A, Malyszczak K, Pyszel K, et al. Physical and psychological impairments of women with upper lymphedema following breast cancer treatment. *Psycho-Oncol*. 2009;*19*:299–305.

3. Fu MR. Breast cancer-related lymphedema: symptoms, diagnosis, risk reduction, and management. *World J Clin Oncol*. 2014;*5*(3):241–247.

4. McLaughlin SA, Bagaria S, Gibson T, et al. Trends in risk reduction practices for the prevention of lymphedema in the first 12 months after breast cancer surgery. *J Am Coll Surg*. 2013;*216*:380–389.

5. Cormier JN, Askew RL, Mungovan KS, et al. Lymphedema beyond breast cancer. *Cancer*. 2010;*116*: 5138–5149

6. Kwan ML, Darbinian J, Schmitz KH, et al. Risk factors for lymphedema in a prospective breast cancer survivorship study: the Pathways Study. *Arch Surg*. 2010;*145*:1055–1063.

7. Fu MR, Rosedale M. Breast cancer survivors' experience of lymphedema related symptoms. *J Pain Symptom Manage*. 2009;*38*(6):849–859.

8. Shih YC, Xu Y, Cormier JN, et al. Incidence, treatment costs, and complications of lymphedema after breast cancer among women of working age: a 2-year follow-up study. *J Clin Oncol*. 2009;*27*(12):2007–2014.

9. Armer JM, Stewart BR. A comparison of four diagnostic criteria for lymphedema in a post-breast cancer population. *Lymphat Res Biol*. 2005;*3*:208–217.

10. Cemal Y, Pusic A, Mehrara BJ. Preventative measures for lymphedema: separating fact from fiction. *J Am Coll Surg*. 2011;*213*(4):543–551.

11. Kwan ML, Cohn JC, Armer JM, et al. Exercise in patients with lymphedema: a systematic review of the contemporary literature. *J Cancer Survivorship*. 2011;*5*(4):320–336.

12. Ridner SH, Fu MR, Wanchai A, et al. Self-management of lymphedema: a systematic review of literature from 2004 to 2011. *Nurs Res*. 2012;*61*(4):291–299.

13. Wanchai A, Beck M, Stewart BR, Armer JM. Management of lymphedema for cancer patients with complex needs. *Semin Oncol Nurs*. 2013;*29*(1):61–65.

14. Lasinski BB, Thrift KM, Squire D, et al. A systematic review of the evidence for complete decongestive therapy in the treatment of lymphedema from 2004 to 2011. *Physic Med Rehabil*. 2012;*4*(8):580–601.

15. Feldman JL, Stout NL, Wanchai A, et al. Intermittent pneumatic compression therapy: a systematic review. *Lymphology*. 2012;*45*(1):13–25.

Chapter 6

Skin Disorders

Pressure Ulcers—Prevention and Management

Barbara M. Bates-Jensen and Sirin Petch

Introduction

Palliative care for skin disorders is a broad area, encompassing prevention and care for chronic wounds such as pressure ulcers, management of malignant wounds and fistulas, and management of stomas. The goals of treatment are to reduce discomfort and pain, manage odor and drainage, and provide for optimal functional capacity. In each area, involvement of the caregiver and family in the plan of care is important. Management of skin disorders involves significant physical care as well as attention to psychological and social care. To meet the needs of the patient and family, access to the multidisciplinary care team is crucial, and consultation by an enterostomal therapy nurse, a certified wound, ostomy, and continence nurse, or a certified wound care nurse is highly desirable.

Because skin disorders are such an important issue in palliative nursing care, the content is covered across two chapters, with Chapter 6 addressing pressure ulcers and Chapter 7 addressing malignant wounds, fistulas, and stomas.

Definition

Pressure ulcers are areas of local tissue trauma that usually develop where soft tissues are compressed between bony prominences and external surfaces for prolonged periods. Mechanical injury to the skin and tissues causes hypoxia and ischemia, leading to tissue necrosis. Caring for the patient with a pressure ulcer can be frustrating for clinicians because of the chronic nature of the wound and because additional time and resources are often invested in the management of these wounds. Further, many family caregivers and health care providers view development of pressure ulcers as an indication of poor care or impending death. Pressure ulcers are painful, care is costly, and treatment costs increase as the severity of the wound increases. Additionally, not all pressure ulcers heal, and many heal slowly, causing a continual drain on caregivers and on financial resources. The chronic nature of a pressure ulcer challenges the health care provider to design more effective treatment plans.

Once a pressure ulcer develops, the usual goals are to manage the wound to support healing. However, some patients will benefit most from a palliative wound care approach. Palliative wound care goals are comfort and limiting the extent or impact of the wound, but without the intent of healing.[1]

Risk Factors for Pressure Ulcers

Pressure ulcers are physical evidence of multiple causative influences. Factors that contribute to pressure ulcer development can be thought of as those that affect the pressure force over the bony prominence and those that affect the tolerance of the tissues to pressure.

- Immobility
- Inactivity
- Sensory loss
- Shear
- Friction
- Moisture
- Incontinence
- Nutritional risk factors
- Age
- Medical conditions and psychological factors
- Environmental resources

Use of Risk Assessment Scales

For practitioners to intervene in a cost-effective way, a method of screening for risk factors is necessary. Several risk assessment instruments are available to clinicians. The most commonly used risk assessment tool for adults in the United States is the Braden Scale for Predicting Pressure Sore Risk.[2] The Braden Scale was developed in 1987 and is composed of six subscales that conceptually reflect degrees of sensory perception, moisture, activity, nutrition, friction and shear, and mobility. All subscales are rated from 1 to 4, except for friction and shear, which is rated from 1 to 3. The subscales may be summed for a total score ranging from 6 to 23. Lower scores indicate lower function and higher risk for development of a pressure ulcer. The cutoff score for hospitalized adults is considered to be 16, with scores of 16 and lower indicating at-risk status.[2] The Braden Scale is the model used in this chapter for prevention of pressure ulcers in patients requiring palliative care.

Regardless of the instrument chosen to evaluate risk status, the clinical relevance is threefold. First, assessment for risk status must occur at frequent intervals. Assessment should be performed at admission to the health care organization (within 24 hours), at predetermined intervals (usually weekly), and whenever a significant change occurs in the patient's general health and status. The second clinical implication is the targeting of specific prevention strategies to identified risk factors. The final clinical implication is for those patients in whom prevention is not successful. For patients with an actual pressure ulcer, the continued monitoring of risk status may prevent further tissue trauma at the wound site and development of additional wound sites.

Prevention of Pressure Ulcers

Prevention strategies are targeted at reducing risk factors and can be focused on eliminating specific risk factors. Early intervention for pressure ulcers is risk factor specific and prophylactic in nature. Prevention is a key element for palliative care.

Eliminating Immobility, Inactivity, and Sensory Loss

Patients who have impaired ability to reposition and who cannot independently change body positions must have local pressure alleviated by any of the following:

- Passive repositioning by caregivers
- Pillow bridging
- Pressure redistribution support surfaces for bed and chair[3]

Reducing Friction and Shear

Measures to reduce friction and shear relate to passive or active movement of the patient. To reduce friction, several interventions are appropriate.

- Providing topical preparations to eliminate or reduce the surface tension between the skin and the bed linen or support surface assists in reducing friction-related injury.
- To lessen friction-induced skin breakdown, appropriate techniques must be used when moving patients so that skin is never dragged across the linens.
- Use of a protective film such as a transparent film dressing or a skin sealant, a protective dressing such as a thin hydrocolloid, or protective padding helps to eliminate the surface contact of the area and decrease the friction between the skin and the linens. Even though heel, ankle, and elbow protectors do nothing to reduce or relieve pressure, they can be effective aids against friction.
- Most shear injury can be eliminated by proper positioning, such as avoidance of the semi-Fowler position and limited use of upright positions (i.e., positions more than 30 degrees inclined).

Maintaining Nutrition

Nutrition is an important element in maintaining healthy skin and tissues. There is a strong relationship between nutrition and pressure ulcer development. The severity of pressure ulceration is correlated with severity of nutritional deficits, especially low protein intake and low serum albumin levels.[4]

Managing Moisture

The preventive interventions related to moisture include general skin care and assessment of incontinence.

General Skin Care

General skin care involves routine skin assessment, incontinence assessment and management, skin hygiene interventions, and measures to maintain skin health. Routine skin assessment involves observation of the patient's skin, with particular attention to bony prominences. Incontinence-associated dermatitis or moisture-associated skin damage is inflammation of the skin that happens when the perineal area is subject to prolonged contact with urine or stool. Objective signs of incontinence-associated dermatitis include erythema, swelling, vesiculation, oozing, crusting, and scaling, with subjective symptoms of tingling, itching, burning, and pain.[5]

Incontinence Assessment

Assessment of incontinence should include history of the incontinence, including patterns of elimination, characteristics of the urinary stream or fecal mass, and sensation of bladder or rectal filling. The physical examination is designed to gather specific information related to bladder or rectal functioning and therefore is limited in scope. A limited neurologic examination should provide data on the mental status and motivation of the patient and caregiver, specific motor skills, and condition of the back and lower extremities. The genitalia and perineal skin are assessed for signs of perineal skin lesions and perineal sensation.

Pressure Ulcer Assessment

The foundation for designing a palliative care plan for the patient with a pressure ulcer is a comprehensive assessment. Comprehensive assessment includes assessment of wound severity, wound status, and the total patient.

- *Wound severity:* Assessment of wound severity refers to the use of a classification system for diagnosing the severity of tissue trauma by determining the tissue layers involved in the wound. Classification systems such as staging pressure ulcers provide communication regarding wound severity and the tissue layers involved in the injury. Table 6.1 presents pressure ulcer staging criteria according to the National Pressure Ulcer Advisory Panel (NPUAP).

Table 6.1 National Pressure Ulcer Advisory Panel Pressure Ulcer Staging Classification

Stage	Definition
Stage I	• Intact skin with nonblanchable redness of a localized area usually over a bony prominence. Darkly pigmented skin may not have visible blanching; its color may differ from the surrounding area. • **Further description:** The area may be painful, firm, soft, warmer, or cooler compared with adjacent tissue. Stage I may be difficult to detect in individuals with dark skin tones. May indicate "at-risk" persons (a heralding sign of risk).
Stage II	• Partial-thickness loss of dermis presenting as a shallow open ulcer with a red-pink wound bed, without slough. May also present as an intact or open/ruptured serum-filled blister. • **Further description:** Presents as a shiny or dry shallow ulcer without slough or bruising.* This stage should not be used to describe skin tears, tape burns, perineal dermatitis, maceration, or excoriation.

(continued)

Table 6.1 (Continued)

Stage	Definition
Stage III	• Full-thickness tissue loss. Subcutaneous fat may be visible, but bone, tendon, and muscle are not exposed. Slough may be present but does not obscure the depth of tissue loss. May include undermining and tunneling.
	• **Further description:**
	The depth of a stage III pressure ulcer varies by anatomic location. The bridge of the nose, ear, occiput, and malleolus do not have subcutaneous tissue, and stage III ulcers can be shallow. In contrast, areas of significant adiposity can develop extremely deep stage III pressure ulcers. Bone and tendon are not visible or directly palpable.
Stage IV	• Full-thickness tissue loss with exposed bone, tendon, or muscle. Slough or eschar may be present on some parts of the wound bed. Often includes undermining and tunneling.
	• **Further description:**
	The depth of a stage IV pressure ulcer varies by anatomic location. The bridge of the nose, ear, occiput, and malleolus do not have subcutaneous tissue, and these ulcers can be shallow. Stage IV ulcers can extend into muscle and/or supporting structures (e.g., fascia, tendon, or joint capsule), making osteomyelitis possible. Exposed bone and tendon are visible or directly palpable.
Unstageable	• Full-thickness tissue loss in which the base of the ulcer is covered by slough (yellow, tan, gray, green, or brown) and/or eschar (tan, brown, or black) in the wound bed.
	• **Further description:**
	Until enough slough and eschar are removed to expose the base of the wound, the true depth, and therefore stage, cannot be determined. Stable (dry, adherent, intact without erythema or fluctuance) eschar on the heels serves as "the body's natural (biologic) cover" and should not be removed.
Suspected deep tissue injury	• Purple or maroon localized area of discolored intact skin or blood-filled blister due to damage of underlying soft tissue from pressure and/or shear. The area may be preceded by tissue that is painful, firm, mushy, boggy, warmer, or cooler compared with adjacent tissue.
	• **Further description:**
	Deep tissue injury may be difficult to detect in individuals with dark skin tones. Evolution may include a thin blister over a dark wound bed. The wound may further evolve and become covered by thin eschar. Evolution may be rapid, exposing additional layers of tissue even with optimal treatment.

*Bruising indicates suspected deep tissue injury.

Adapted from National Pressure Ulcer Advisory Panel and European Pressure Ulcer Advisory Panel. *Prevention and Treatment of Pressure Ulcers: Clinical Practice Guideline.* Washington DC: National Pressure Ulcer Advisory Panel; 2009.

- *Wound status:* Pressure ulcer assessment is the base for maintaining and evaluating the therapeutic plan of care. Assessment of wound status involves evaluation of multiple wound characteristics. Initial assessment and follow-up assessments at regular intervals to monitor progress or deterioration of the sore are necessary to determine the effectiveness of the treatment plan. Adequate assessment is important even when the goal of care is comfort, not healing. The assessment data enable clinicians to communicate clearly about a patient's pressure ulcer, provide for continuity in the plan of care, and allow evaluation of treatment modalities. Assessment of wound status should be performed weekly and whenever a significant change is noted in the wound.

- *Wound characteristics:* Adequate initial wound assessment should encompass a composite of wound characteristics, which forms a base for differential diagnosis, therapeutic intervention, and future reassessment comparisons. The indices for wound assessment include all of the following: location, size of ulcer, depth of tissue involvement, stage or classification, condition of wound edges, presence of undermining or tunneling, necrotic tissue characteristics, exudate characteristics, surrounding tissue conditions, and wound healing characteristics of granulation tissue and epithelialization. Wound characteristics of concern for the palliative care patient include wound edges, undermining and tunneling, necrotic tissue characteristics, exudate characteristics, and surrounding tissue conditions.

Total Patient Assessment

Comprehensive assessment includes assessment of the total patient as well as of wound severity and wound status. Generally, diagnosis and management of the wound are best accomplished within the context of the whole person. Comprehensive assessment includes a focused history and physical examination, attention to specific laboratory and diagnostic tests, and a pain assessment. Box 6.1 presents an overview of assessment for the patient with a pressure ulcer.

It is important to obtain a focused history and physical examination as part of the initial assessment. The patient history determines which relevant systems reviews are needed in the physical examination. The goals for treatment and the direction of care (e.g., curative with a goal of wound closure, palliative with a goal of reduced wound pain) can be determined with, at a minimum, the following patient history information: reason for admission to care facility or agency; expectations and perceptions about wound healing; psychological, social, cultural, and economic history; presence of medical comorbidities; current wound status; and previous management strategies.

Pressure Ulcer Management

Pressure ulcer management should be based on clinical practice guidelines. The NPUAP in conjunction with the European Pressure Ulcer Advisory Panel presented updated pressure ulcer guidelines in 2009,[3] which include specific guidelines for palliative care and pain management. The general NPUAP palliative care guidelines are listed in Box 6.2. Guidelines for palliative care include the following:

Box 6.1 Bates-Jensen Wound Assessment Tool: Instructions for Use

General Guidelines

Fill out the attached rating sheet to assess a wound's status after reading the definitions and methods of assessment described below. Evaluate once a week and whenever a change occurs in the wound. Rate according to each item by picking the response that best describes the wound and entering that score in the item score column for the appropriate date. When you have rated the wound on all items, determine the total score by adding together the 13-item scores. The *higher* the total score, the more severe the wound status. Plot the total score on the Wound Status Continuum to determine progress. If the wound has healed/resolved, score items 1, 2, 3, and 4 as =0.

Specific Instructions

1. **Size**: Use a ruler to measure the longest and widest aspect of the wound surface in centimeters; multiply length × width. Score as =0 if wound healed/resolved.
2. **Depth**: Pick the depth, or thickness, most appropriate to the wound using these additional descriptions, score as =0 if the wound has healed/resolved:
   1 = tissues damaged but no break in skin surface
   2 = superficial, abrasion, blister, or shallow crater; even with and/or elevated above skin surface (e.g., hyperplasia)
   3 = deep crater with or without undermining of adjacent tissue
   4 = visualization of tissue layers not possible because of necrosis
   5 = supporting structures include tendon, joint capsule
3. **Edges**: Score as = 0 if wound has healed/resolved. Use this guide:

Indistinct, diffuse	= unable to clearly distinguish wound outline
Attached	= even or flush with wound base, *no* sides or walls present; flat
Not attached	= sides or walls *are* present; floor or base of wound is deeper than edge
Rolled under, thickened	= soft to firm and flexible to touch
Hyperkeratosis	= callous-like tissue formation around wound and at edges
Fibrotic, scarred	= hard, rigid to touch

4. **Undermining**: Score as = 0 if wound has healed/resolved. Assess by inserting a cotton-tipped applicator under the wound edge; advance it as far as it will go without using undue force; raise the tip of the applicator so that it may be seen or felt on the surface of the skin; mark the surface with a pen; measure the distance from the mark on the skin to the edge of the wound. Continue process around the wound. Then use a transparent metric measuring guide with concentric circles divided into 4 (25%) pie-shaped quadrants to help determine percentage of wound involved.

(continued)

Box 6.1 (Continued)

5. **Necrotic Tissue Type**: Pick the type of necrotic tissue that is *predominant* in the wound according to color, consistency, and adherence using this guide:

White/gray nonviable tissue	= may appear prior to wound opening; skin surface is white or gray
Nonadherent, yellow slough	= thin, mucinous substance; scattered throughout wound bed; easily separated from wound tissue
Loosely adherent, yellow slough	= thick, stringy, clumps of debris; attached to wound tissue
Adherent, soft, black eschar	= soggy tissue; strongly attached to tissue in center or base of wound
Firmly adherent, hard/black eschar	= firm, crusty tissue; strongly attached to wound base *and* edges (like a hard scab)

6. **Necrotic Tissue Amount**: Use a transparent metric measuring guide with concentric circles divided into 4 (25%) pie-shaped quadrants to help determine percentage of wound involved.

7. **Exudate Type**: Some dressings interact with wound drainage to produce a gel or trap liquid. Before assessing exudate type, gently cleanse wound with normal saline or water. Pick the exudate type that is *predominant* in the wound according to color and consistency, using this guide:

Bloody	= thin, bright red
Serosanguineous	= thin, watery pale red to pink
Serous	= thin, watery, clear
Purulent	= thin or thick, opaque tan to yellow or green, may have offensive odor

8. **Exudate Amount**: Use a transparent metric measuring guide with concentric circles divided into 4 (25%) pie-shaped quadrants to determine percentage of dressing involved with exudate. Use this guide:

None	= wound tissues dry
Scant	= wound tissues moist; no measurable exudate
Small	= wound tissues wet; moisture evenly distributed in wound; drainage involves ≤25% dressing
Moderate	= wound tissues saturated; drainage may or may not be evenly distributed in wound; drainage involves >25% to ≤75% dressing
Large	= wound tissues bathed in fluid; drainage freely expressed; may or may not be evenly distributed in wound; drainage involves >75% of dressing

(continued)

Box 6.1 (Continued)

9. **Skin Color Surrounding Wound**: Assess tissues within 4 cm of wound edge. Dark-skinned persons show the colors "bright red" and "dark red" as a deepening of normal ethnic skin color or a purple hue. As healing occurs in dark-skinned persons, the new skin is pink and may never darken.

10. **Peripheral Tissue Edema and Induration**: Assess tissues within 4 cm of wound edge. Nonpitting edema appears as skin that is shiny and taut. Identify pitting edema by firmly pressing a finger down into the tissues and waiting 5 seconds; on release of pressure, tissues fail to resume previous position, and an indentation appears. Induration is abnormal firmness of tissues with margins. Assess by gently pinching the tissues. Induration results in an inability to pinch the tissues. Use a transparent metric measuring guide to determine how far edema or induration extends beyond the wound.

11. **Granulation Tissue**: Granulation tissue is the growth of small blood vessels and connective tissue to fill in full-thickness wounds. Tissue is healthy when bright, beefy red, shiny, and granular with a velvety appearance. Poor vascular supply appears as pale pink or blanched to dull, dusky red color.

12. **Epithelialization**: Epithelialization is the process of epidermal resurfacing and appears as pink or red skin. In partial-thickness wounds, it can occur throughout the wound bed as well as from the wound edges. In full-thickness wounds, it occurs from the edges only. Use a transparent metric measuring guide with concentric circles divided into 4 (25%) pie-shaped quadrants to help determine percentage of wound involved and to measure the distance the epithelial tissue extends into the wound.

© 2006 Barbara Bates-Jensen.

Box 6.2 National Pressure Ulcer Advisory Panel Recommended Palliative Care Pressure Ulcer Guidelines

1. Assess the risk for new pressure ulcer development by using a validated risk assessment tool.

2. Reposition the individual at periodic intervals in accordance with the individual's wishes.

3. Strive to maintain adequate nutrition and hydration compatible with the individual's condition and wishes. Adequate nutrition is often not attainable if the individual is unable or refuses to eat.

4. Maintain skin integrity to the extent possible.

5. Set treatment goals that are consistent with the values and goals of the individual.

6. The goal for the palliative care individual with a pressure ulcer is often to enhance quality of life, even if the pressure ulcer cannot or does not lead to closure.

(continued)

Box 6.2 (Continued)

7. Assess the individual initially and whenever there is a change in factors placing the individual at risk.

8. Assess the pressure ulcer initially and weekly and document findings. Assess the pressure ulcer with each dressing change.

9. Assess the impact of the pressure ulcer on quality of life of the patient and family.

10. Manage the pressure ulcer and peri-wound area on a regular basis.

11. Control wound odor.

12. Assess wound pain.

13. Assess resources.

- Repositioning the individual at periodic intervals in accordance with the individual's wishes
- Striving to maintain adequate nutrition and hydration compatible with the individual's condition and wishes, with the understanding that adequate nutrition is often not attainable if the individual is unable or refuses to eat
- Managing the pressure ulcer and peri-wound skin on a routine, regular basis
- Controlling wound odor
- Reducing wound pain

Patient and Caregiver Teaching Guidelines

Patient and caregiver instruction in self-care must be individualized according to specific pressure ulcer development risk factors, individual learning styles and coping mechanisms, and the ability of the patient or caregiver to perform procedures. In teaching prevention guidelines to caregivers, it is particularly important to use return demonstration to evaluate learning. Observing the caregiver perform turning maneuvers, repositioning, managing incontinence, and providing general skin care can be enlightening and provides a context in which the clinician supports and follows up education. In palliative care, it is important to include the reasons for specific actions, such as the continuation of some level of turning and repositioning to prevent further tissue damage and lessen discomfort from additional wounds. The patient and family should be informed about pressure ulcer development at the end of life, and the information should be presented so that there is understanding that not all pressure ulcers are avoidable. If a pressure ulcer develops, reminding the patient and caregiver of the care that has been provided and that the pressure ulcer is not a reflection of poor care is important to help allay any feeling of guilt.

Conclusion

Poorly managed pressure ulcers can increase pain and suffering in those with a chronic debilitating illness. Although preventive measure in patients identified as at risk for developing such pressure ulcers can be effective, some patients do develop pressure ulcers that require expert nursing management. Expert nursing management includes instituting preventive measures to preserve intact skin, obtaining and maintaining a clean wound, management of exudate and odor, and prevention of complications such as a superimposed wound infection. Because many dying and chronically ill debilitated patients are cared for at home, educating family members about the development of pressure ulcers and involving family caregivers in the plan of care are critical. This is especially true because many caregivers view pressure ulcers as a reflection of poor care, and in reality, pressure ulcer development in persons at the end of life or in persons with certain comorbidites may be unavoidable even with the best care.

References

1. Hendrichova I, Castellie M, Mastroianni C, et al. Pressure ulcers in cancer palliative care patients. *Palliat Med.* 2010;*24*(7):669–673.

2. Bergstrom N, Demuth PJ, Braden BJ. A clinical trial of the Braden Scale for Predicting Pressure Sore Risk. *Nurs Clin North Am.* 1987;*22*:417–428.

3. National Pressure Ulcer Advisory Panel and European Pressure Ulcer Advisory Panel. *Prevention and Treatment of Pressure Ulcers: Clinical Practice Guideline.* Washington DC: National Pressure Ulcer Advisory Panel, 2009.

4. Iizaka S, Okuwa M, Sugama J, Sanada H. The impact of malnutrition and nutrition-related factors on the development and severity of pressure ulcers in older patients receiving home care. *Clin Nutr.* 2009;*29*(1):47–53.

5. Gray M, Bliss DZ, Doughty DB, et al. Incontinence-associated dermatitis: a consensus. *J Wound Ostomy Continence Nurs.* 2007;*34*:45–54.

Chapter 7

Skin Disorders

Malignant Wounds, Fistulas, and Stomas

Susie Seaman and Barbara M. Bates-Jensen

Malignant Wounds

Introduction

Malignant wounds, also known in the literature as fungating tumors, tumor necrosis, ulcerative malignant wounds, or fungating malignant wounds, present both a physical and an emotional challenge for the patient, caregiver, and clinician. These wounds are frequently associated with pain, odor, bleeding, and an unsightly appearance. They may be a blow to self-esteem and may cause social isolation just when the patient needs more time with loved ones. The goals in the care of patients with malignant wounds include managing wound exudate, odor, bleeding, and pain; preventing infection; and promoting the emotional welfare of the patient and family.

Assessment

Ongoing comprehensive assessment of the patient and malignant wound facilitates formulation of an appropriate treatment plan, allows for adjustment of the treatment plan as findings change, and promotes recognition of wound complications. Specifically, wound location, size, appearance, exudate, and odor and the condition of the surrounding skin guide local therapy. Associated symptoms should be noted so that appropriate measures can be taken to provide comfort. The potential for serious complications such as hemorrhage, vessel compression or obstruction, or airway obstruction should be noted so that the caregiver can be educated regarding their palliative management. Table 7.1 presents highlights for the assessment of malignant wounds and associated rationale.

Management

The goals of care for patients with malignant wounds include control of infection and odor, management of exudate, prevention and control of bleeding, and management of pain.[1-4] In determining the appropriate treatment regimen, the abilities of the caregiver must also be considered.

Table 7.1 Assessment of Malignant Wounds

Assessment	Rationale
Wound Location	
Is mobility impaired?	Consider occupational therapy referral to facilitate activities of daily living
Located near wrinkled or flat skin?	Affects dressing selection Affects dressing fixation
Able to hide from public view?	Affects psychological coping
Wound Appearance	
Size: length, width, depth, undermining, deep structure exposure	Affects dressing selection, provides information on deterioration or response to palliative treatment
Fungating or ulcerative	Affects dressing selection and fixation
Percentage of viable vs. necrotic tissue	Need for cleansing or debridement
Tissue friability and bleeding	Need for nonadherent dressings and other measures to control bleeding
Presence of odor	Need for odor-reducing strategies
Presence of fistula	Possible need for pouching
Exudate amount	Affects dressing selection
Wound colonized or clinically infected	Need for local versus systemic care
Surrounding Skin	
Erythematous	Infection or tumor extension
Fragile or denuded	Impacts dressing type and fixation
Nodular	Tumor extension or metastasis
Macerated	Need for improved exudate management
Radiation-related skin damage	Need for topical care of skin, affects dressing fixation
Symptoms	
Deep pain: aching, stabbing, continuous	Need to adjust systemic analgesia
Superficial pain: burning, stinging, may be associated only with dressing changes	Need for topical analgesia and rapid-onset, short-acting analgesics
Pruritus	Related to dressings? If not, may need systemic antipruritic medications
Potential for Serious Complications	
Lesion is near major blood vessels: potential for hemorrhage	Need for education of patient and family about palliative management of severe bleeding
Lesion is near major blood vessels: potential for vessel compression or obstruction	Need for education of patient and family about palliative management of severe swelling and pain, possible tissue necrosis
Lesion is near airway: potential for obstruction	Need for education of patient and family about palliative management of airway obstruction

Infection and Odor Control

Control of infection and odor is achieved by controlling local bacterial colonization with wound cleansing, wound debridement, and use of local antimicrobial agents. Because malignant wounds are frequently associated with necrotic tissue and odor, wound cleansing is essential to remove necrotic debris, decrease bacterial counts, and thus reduce odor.

If the lesion is not very friable, the patient may be able to shower. This not only provides for local cleansing but also gives the added psychological benefit of helping the patient to feel clean.

If there is friable tissue (i.e., tissue that bleeds easily with minimal trauma) or the patient is not able to shower, the nurse or caregiver should gently irrigate the wound with normal saline or a commercial wound cleanser.

Skin and incontinence cleansers, which contain mild soaps and antibacterial ingredients used in bathing, can be very effective at controlling local bacterial colonization and odor. As long as they do not cause burning, they may be sprayed directly on the wound. If pain and burning occur with use of skin cleansers in the wound, these cleansers should be used only on the surrounding skin.

Topical antimicrobial agents such as hydrogen peroxide, sodium hypochlorite (Dakin's solution), and povidone iodine are recommended by some authors; however, their use should be weighed against the potential negative effects of local pain, skin irritation, wound desiccation with subsequent pain and bleeding on dressing removal, and unpleasant odor associated with Dakin's and povidone iodine.[5]

Newer antimicrobial wound cleansers containing polyhexamethylene biguanide (PHMB) may help decrease bacterial colonization while minimizing toxicity to healthy cells.[5-8] Gauze soaked with a PHMB cleanser can be applied to the wound for 15 minutes before new dressing application for optimal decolonization.

Odor is by far the most difficult management aspect of treating malignant wounds and is frequently the most distressing complaint that affected patients have. The literature supports use of topical metronidazole, which has a wide range of activity against anaerobic bacteria, to control wound odor.[9] Topical therapy is available by crushing metronidazole tablets in sterile water and creating either a 0.5% solution (5 mg/mL) or a 1% solution (10 mg/mL). This may be used as a wound irrigant, or gauze may be saturated with the solution and packed into wound cavities. Care must be taken not to allow the gauze packing to desiccate because dressing adherence may lead to bleeding and pain. An easy, effective alternative to metronidazole solution is metronidazole 0.75% gel, which is applied in a thin layer to the entire wound.

In low exudate wounds in which dressing adherence is a concern, the gel should be covered with a nonadherent contact layer, and then absorbent dressings such as gauze or ABD pads should be applied. In more heavily draining wounds, a nonadherent contact layer may not be necessary, and the absorbent dressings can be applied directly to the wound. For optimal odor control, dressings should be changed daily, and more often for high levels of exudate that soak through the bandage.

Systemic use of metronidazole should be employed only in patients with invasive infection, not in those with local bacterial colonization.

There are dressings that may also help decrease bacterial colonization and odor in malignant wounds.[8] Charcoal dressings, which absorb and trap odor, are available as either primary or secondary bandages.

Any dressing that decreases bacterial counts in a wound has the potential to decrease odor. Silver has broad-spectrum activity against microorganisms found in wounds.[10] Silver-based dressings are available in multiple different types, including alginates, hydrocolloids, hydrogels, hydrofibers, foams, contact layers, and mesh gauze.

Less conventional methods of odor management are also available. Environmental deodorizers such as cat litter or charcoal briquettes can be placed under the bed to help reduce room odor for patients at home.[3] Use of peppermint oil or other aromatherapy products, applied below the nostril or near the bed, may help mask the odor. Odor-eliminating room sprays are more effective than room deodorant sprays and can be used before and after wound care to reduce the odor associated with wound exposure.

Clinical infection, as evidenced by erythema, induration, increased pain and exudate, leukocytosis, and fever, should be treated with systemic antibiotics. Cultures should be used to identify infecting organisms after the wound is diagnosed with an infection based on clinical signs; cultures should not be taken routinely to diagnose infection. Because of the local inflammatory effects of the tumor, wounds may have many of the same signs as infection, so the clinician must be discriminating in differentiating between the two. A complete blood count, assessing the white cell count and differential, may be helpful in guiding assessment and therapy. It is crucial to avoid treating patients with oral antibiotics if the wound is only colonized and not infected, to prevent side effects and emergence of resistant organisms.

Management of Exudate

Because of the inflammation and edema commonly associated with malignant wounds, there tends to be significant exudate. Dressings should be chosen to conceal and collect exudate and odor. This is essential because a patient who experiences unexpected drainage on clothing or bedding may suffer significant feelings of distress and loss of control. Specialty dressings, such as foams, alginates, or starch copolymers, are notably more expensive than gauze pads or cotton-based absorbent pads. However, if such dressings reduce the overall cost by reducing the need for frequent dressing changes, they may be cost-effective. Table 7.2 summarizes dressing considerations with malignant wounds.

Controlling Bleeding

The viable tissue in a malignant wound may be very friable, bleeding with even minimal manipulation. Prevention is the best therapy for controlling bleeding. Prevention involves use of a gentle hand in dressing removal and thoughtful attention to the use of nonadherent dressings or moist wound dressings. On wounds with a low amount of exudate, the use of hydrogel sheets, or amorphous hydrogels under a nonadherent contact layer, may keep the wound moist and prevent dressing adherence. Even highly exudating wounds may require a nonadherent contact layer to allow for atraumatic dressing removal.

Table 7.2 Dressing Choices for Malignant Wounds

Type of Wound and Goals of Care	Dressing Choice
Low Exudate	
Maintain moist environment Prevent dressing adherence and bleeding	Nonadherent contact layers • Adaptic (Systagenix) • Adaptic Touch (Systagenix) • Conformant 2 (Smith & Nephew) • Dermanet (DeRoyal) • Mepitel One (Mölnlycke) • Mepilex Transfer (Mölnlycke) • Petrolatum gauze (numerous manufacturers) • Restore Contact Layer (Hollister) • Tegaderm Contact (3M Health Care) Amorphous hydrogels Sheet hydrogels Hydrocolloids: contraindicated with fragile surrounding skin, may increase odor Semipermeable films: contraindicated with fragile surrounding skin
High Exudate	
Absorb and contain exudate Prevent dressing adherence in areas of lesion with decreased exudate	Alginates Foams Starch copolymers Gauze Soft cotton pads Menstrual pads (excessive exudate)
Malodorous Wounds	
Wound cleansing (see text) Reduce or eliminate odor	Charcoal dressings Topical metronidazole (see text) Iodosorb Gel (Healthpoint): iodine-based, may cause burning Prontosan Gel (B. Braun) Honey-based dressings Silver-based dressings

If dressings adhere to the wound on attempted removal, they should be soaked away with normal saline to lessen the trauma to the wound bed. If bleeding does occur, the first intervention should be direct pressure applied for 10 to 15 minutes. Local ice packs may also assist in controlling bleeding. If pressure alone is ineffective, several other options exist.[11]

- Application of an alginate dressing or sucralfate paste (1 g sucralfate tablet crushed in 5 mL water-soluble gel) may stop mild bleeding.
- Gauze soaked with 1:1000 epinephrine applied to the wound may control bleeding but can lead to local tissue necrosis. Other local vasoconstrictive agents may be used, including topical cocaine or oxymetazoline spray.[11]
- Small bleeding points can be controlled with silver nitrate sticks.
- As an alternative, use of topical, absorbable hemostatic agents made from gelatin, collagen, and/or oxidized regenerated cellulose (e.g., Gelfoam, Surgicel, Promogran) may be appropriate but are costly. Moh's paste, a chemical fixative applied topically to the wound, has been shown to be successful at controlling bleeding in gynecologic and breast cancer tumors. Caution must be used to avoid excessive tissue damage, peri-wound dermatitis, and pain associated with this treatment.

Pain Management

Several types of pain are associated with tumor malignant wounds: deep pain, neuropathic pain, and superficial pain related to procedures. Deep pain should be managed by premedication before dressing changes. Opioids for preprocedural medication may be needed, and rapid-onset, short-acting analgesics may be especially useful for those already receiving other long-acting opioid medication. For management of superficial pain related to procedures, topical lidocaine or benzocaine may be helpful.[12] These local analgesics may be applied to the wound immediately after dressing removal, with wound care delayed until adequate local anesthesia is obtained. Ice packs used before or after wound care may also be helpful to reduce pain. Another option for topical analgesia is the use of topical opioids, which bind to peripheral opioid receptors.[13] Topical opioids may be a viable adjunct to systemic analgesia in the care of patients with malignant wounds.

Promotion of Patient and Caregiver Welfare Through Education

Dealing with a cancer diagnosis is traumatic enough without the added physical and psychological burden of a malignant wound. Assisting the patient and the caregiver to cope with the distressing symptoms of the malignant wound so that odor and bleeding are managed, exudate is contained, and pain is alleviated will improve the quality of life for these patients and contribute to the goal of satisfactory psychological well-being. Education must include realistic goals for the wound. In these patients, the goal of complete wound healing is seldom achievable; however, quality of life can be maintained even as the wound degenerates. Continual education and reevaluation of the effectiveness of the treatment plan are essential to maintaining quality of life for those suffering from a malignant wound.

Fistulas

Introduction

A fistula is an abnormal passage or opening between two or more body organs or spaces. The most frequently involved organs are the skin and either the bladder or the digestive tract, although fistulas can occur between many other body organs and spaces. Often, the organs involved and the location of the fistula in difficult anatomic areas or open abdominal wounds influence management methods and complicate care. For example, fistulas involving the small bowel and the vaginal vault and those involving the esophagus and skin create extreme challenges in care related to both the location and the organs involved in the fistula. Factors that inhibit fistula closure include complete disruption of bowel continuity, distal obstruction, presence of a foreign body in the fistula tract, an epithelium-lined tract contiguous with the skin, presence of cancer, previous radiation, and Crohn's disease. The presence of any of these factors can be deleterious for spontaneous closure of a fistula. The goals of management for fistula care involve containment of effluent, management of odor, comfort, and protection of the surrounding skin and tissues.

Assessment

Assessment of the fistula involves assessment of the source, surrounding skin, output, and fluid and electrolyte status. Evaluation of the fistula source may involve diagnostic tests such as radiographs to determine the exact structures involved in the fistula tract. Assessment of the fistula source involves evaluation of fistula output, or effluent, for odor, color, consistency, pH, and amount. These characteristics provide clues to the origin of the output. Fistulas with highly odorous output are likely to originate in the colon or may be related to cancerous lesions. Fistula output with less odor may have a small bowel origin. The color of fistula output also provides clues to the source: clear or white output is typical of esophageal fistulas, green output is usual of fistulas originating from the gastric area, and light brown or tan output may indicate small bowel sources. Small bowel output is typically thin and watery to thick and pasty in consistency, whereas colonic fistulas have output with a pasty to a soft consistency. The volume of output is often an indication of the source. For small bowel fistulas, output is typically high, with volumes ranging from 500 to 3000 mL over 24 hours, for low-output and high-output fistulas, respectively. Esophageal fistula output may be as high as 1000 mL over 24 hours. Fistulas can be classified according to output, with those producing less than 500 mL over 24 hours classified as low output and those producing greater volumes classified as high output.

The anatomic orifice location, proximity of the orifice to bony prominences, regularity and stability of the surrounding skin, number of fistula openings, and level at which the fistula orifice exits onto the skin influence treatment options. Fistulas may be classified according to the organs involved and the location of the opening of the fistula orifice. Fistulas with openings from one internal body organ to another (e.g., from small bowel to bladder, from bladder to vagina) are internal fistulas; those with cutaneous involvement (e.g., small bowel to skin) are external fistulas.

Assessment of fluid and electrolyte balance is essential because of the risk for imbalance in both. In particular, the patient with a small bowel fistula is at high risk for fluid volume deficit or dehydration and metabolic acidosis due to the loss of large volumes of alkaline small bowel contents. Significant losses of sodium and potassium are common with small bowel fistulas. Laboratory values should be monitored frequently. Evaluation for signs of fluid volume deficit is also recommended.

Management

Wherever anatomically possible, the fistula should be managed with an ostomy pouching technique. The surrounding skin should be cleansed with warm water without soap or antiseptics; skin barrier paste should then be used to fill uneven skin surfaces so that a flat surface is created to apply the pouch. Pediatric pouches are often smaller and more flexible and may be useful for hard-to-pouch areas where flexibility is needed, such as the neck for esophageal fistulas. Pouches must be emptied frequently, at least when one-third to one-half full. There are several wound drainage pouching systems on the market that allow for visualization and direct access to the fistula through a valve or door that can be opened and closed. These wound management pouches are available in large sizes and often work well for abdominal fistulas. Pouching of the fistula allows for odor control (many fistulas are quite malodorous), containment of output, and protection of the surrounding skin from damage. Gauze dressings with or without charcoal filters may be used if the output from the fistula is less than 250 mL over 24 hours and is not severely offensive in odor. Colostomy caps (small closed-end pouches) can be useful for low-output fistulas that continue to be odorous.

There are specific pouching techniques that are useful in complex fistula management, including troughing, saddlebagging, and bridging.[14] These techniques are particularly helpful when dealing with fistulas that occur in wounds, most commonly the small bowel fistula that develops in the open abdominal wound.

Troughing is useful for fistulas that occur in the posterior aspect of large abdominal wounds. The skin surrounding the wound and fistula should be lined with a skin barrier wafer and the edge nearest the wound sealed with skin barrier paste. Then, thin film dressings are applied over the top or anterior aspect of the wound, down to the fistula orifice and the posterior aspect of the wound. Finally, a cut-to-fit ostomy pouch is used to pouch the opening in the thin film dressing at the fistula orifice. Wound exudate drains from the anterior portion of the wound (under the thin film dressing) to the posterior portion of the wound and out into the ostomy pouch, along with fistula output. The trough technique does not prevent fistula output from contaminating the wound site.

The bridging technique prevents fistula output from contaminating the wound site and allows for a unique wound dressing to be applied to the wound site. Bridging is appropriate for fistulas that occur in the posterior aspect of large abdominal wounds, where it is important to contain fistula output away from the wound site. Using small pieces of skin barrier wafers, the clinician builds a "bridge" by consecutively layering the skin barriers together until the skin barrier has the appearance of a wedge or bridge and is the same height as the depth of the wound. With the use of a skin barrier paste, the skin barrier wedge is adhered to the wound bed (it does not harm the healthy tissues of the wound bed), next to the fistula opening. An ostomy pouch is then cut to fit the fistula opening, using the wedge or bridge as a portion of intact surrounding skin to adhere the pouch. The anterior aspect of the wound may then be dressed with the dressing of choice.

Saddlebagging is used for multiple fistulas, if it is important to keep the output from each fistula separated and the fistula orifices are close together. Two cut-to-fit ostomy pouches (or more for more fistulas) are used. The fistula openings are cut on the back of the pouch, off-center, or as far to the side as possible, and the second pouch is cut to fit the next fistula, off-center, or as far to the other side as possible. The skin is cleansed with warm water, and skin barrier paste is applied around the orifices. Ostomy pouches are applied and, where they contact each other (down the middle), they are affixed or adhered to each other in a "saddlebag" fashion. Multiple fistulas can also be managed with one ostomy pouching system that accommodates the multiple openings. Consultation with an enterostomal therapy (ET) nurse or ostomy nurse is extremely advantageous in these cases.

Another method of managing fistulas is by a closed suction wound drainage system. After the wound is cleansed with normal saline, the fenestrated Jackson-Pratt drain is placed in the wound, on top of a moistened gauze that has been opened up to line the wound bed (primary contact layer); a second fluffed wet gauze is placed over the drain, and the surrounding skin is prepared with a skin sealant. Next, the entire site is covered with a thin film dressing, which is crimped around the tube of the drain where it exits the wound. The tube exit site is filled with skin barrier paste, and the drain is connected to low continuous wall suction; the connection site may need to be adjusted and may require use of a small "Christmas tree" connector or device and tape to secure it.

Negative-pressure wound therapy (NPWT) devices present an easier method of closed suction and have also been used for fistula management.[15] In certain circumstances, NPWT may help to promote healing in wounds with an enteric fistula. Candidates must have a fistula that has been examined or explored, and the fistula opening must be readily visualized and accessible. The patient must be receiving nothing by mouth, on total parenteral nutrition with fistula effluent that is thin to viscous.

Pouches to contain the fistula output usually assist in containing odor as well. If odor continues to be problematic with an intact pouching system, internal body deodorants such as bismuth subgallate, charcoal compositions, or peppermint oil may be helpful. Taking care to change the pouch in a well-ventilated room also helps with odor. If odor is caused by anaerobic bacteria, use of 400 mg metronidazole orally three times a day may be helpful. Management of high-output fistulas may be improved with administration of octreotide 300 mcg subcutaneously over 24 hours.

Nutrition management and fluid and electrolyte maintenance are essential for adequate fistula care. Fluid and nutritional requirements may be greatly increased with fistulas, and there are difficulties with fistulas that involve the gastrointestinal system. As a general guideline, the intestinal system should be used whenever possible for nutritional support. The specific goals of fluid and electrolyte and nutritional support for fistula management must be discussed with the patient and family in view of the palliative nature of the overall care plan.

Patient and Caregiver Education

Patient and caregiver teaching first involves adequate assessment of the self-care ability of the patient and of the caregiver's abilities. The patient and caregiver must be taught the management method for the fistula, including pouching techniques, how to empty the pouch, odor control methods, and strategies for increasing fluid and nutritional intake. Many of the pouching techniques used to manage fistulas are complicated and may require continual surveillance by an expert such as an ET nurse or ostomy nurse.

Palliative Stoma Care

Introduction

The significance of palliative care for an individual with a stoma is to improve well-being during this critical time and to attain the best quality of life possible. In regard to the stoma, palliative care is achieved by restoring the most efficient management plan and providing optimal functional capacity. It is essential to involve the family in the plan of care and to provide care to the extent of the patient's wishes.

Management of the ostomy includes physical care as well as psychological and social care. To meet the needs of the patient and family, access to the multidisciplinary care team is crucial. This team may include the ET nurse, physicians such as the surgeon and oncologist, a nutritionist, and social service personnel. The urinary or fecal stoma can be managed (by the ET nurse) to incorporate the needs and goals of both the patient and the caregiver and to provide the highest quality of life possible.

Types of Diversion

The three types of diversion created with a stoma as the outlet for urine or stool are the ileoconduit (urinary output), the ileostomy (fecal output), and the colostomy (fecal output). Construction of any of these diversions requires the person to wear an external appliance to collect the output.

Ileoconduit

The ileoconduit is the primary method for diverting urinary flow in the absence of bladder function. This procedure involves isolation of a section of the terminal ileum. The proximal end is closed, and the distal end is brought out through an opening in the abdominal wall at a site selected before surgery. The ileal segment is sutured to the skin, creating a stoma. The ureters are implanted into the ileal segment, urine flows into the conduit, and peristalsis propels the urine out through the stoma. An external appliance is worn to collect the urine; it is emptied when the pouch is one-third to one-half full, or approximately every 4 hours.

Ileostomy

The ileostomy is created to divert stool away from the large intestine, typically using the terminal ileum. The stoma is created by bringing the distal end of the ileum through an opening surgically created in the abdominal wall and suturing it to the skin. The output is usually a soft, unformed to semiformed stool. Approximately 600 to 800 mL/day is eliminated. An external appliance is worn to collect the fecal material; it is emptied when the bag is one-third to one-half full, usually four to six times per day. An ileostomy may be temporary or permanent. A temporary ileostomy usually is created when the colon needs time to heal or rest, such as after colon surgery or a colon obstruction. A permanent ileostomy is necessary if the entire colon, rectum, and anus have been surgically removed, such as in colorectal cancer or Crohn's disease.

Colostomy

The colostomy is created proximal to the affected segment of the colon or rectum. A colostomy may be temporary or permanent. There are three sections of the colon: the ascending, transverse, and descending colon. The section of colon used to create the stoma determines in part the location and the consistency of output, which may affect the nutritional and hydration status of the individual at critical times. The ascending colon stoma usually is created on the right midquadrant of the abdomen, and the output is a semiformed stool. The transverse stoma is created in the upper quadrants and is the largest stoma created; the output is usually a semiformed to formed stool. The descending colon stoma most closely mirrors the activity of normal bowel function; it usually is located in the lower left quadrant.

The stoma is created by bringing the distal end of the colon through an opening surgically created in the abdominal wall and suturing it to the skin. An external appliance is worn to collect the fecal material; it is emptied when the bag is one-third to one-half full, usually one or two times per day. A second option for management is irrigation, to regulate the bowel. The patient is taught to instill 600 to 1000 mL of lukewarm tap water through the stoma, using a cone-shaped irrigation apparatus. This creates bowel distention, stimulating peristaltic activity and therefore elimination within 30 to 45 minutes. Repetition of this process over time induces bowel dependence on the stimulus, reducing the spillage of stool between irrigations. The elimination process after initial evacuation is suppressed for 24 to 48 hours.

Assessment

Stoma Characteristics

Viability of the stoma is assessed by its color. This should be checked regularly, especially in the early postoperative period. Normal color of the stoma is deep pink to deep red. The intestinal stomal tissue can be compared with the mucosal lining of the mouth. Stoma edema is normal in the early postoperative period as a result of surgical manipulation. This should not interfere with stoma functioning, but a larger opening will need to be cut in the appliance to prevent pressure or constriction of the stoma. Most stomas decrease by 4 to 6 weeks after surgery, with minor changes over 1 year. Teaching the individual to continue to measure the stoma with each change of appliance should alleviate the problem of wearing an appliance with an aperture too large for the stoma. The stoma needs only a space one-eighth of an inch in diameter to allow for expansion during peristalsis.

Stoma herniation occurs when the bowel moves through the muscle defect created at the time of stoma formation and into the subcutaneous tissue.

The hernia usually reduces spontaneously when the patient lies in a supine position, as a result of decreased intraabdominal pressure. Problems associated with the formation of a peristomal hernia are increased difficulty with ostomy pouch adherence and possible bowel strangulation and obstruction.

Stoma prolapse occurs as a result of a weakened abdominal wall caused by abdominal distention, formation of a loop stoma, or a large aperture in the abdominal wall. The prolapse is a telescoping of the intestine through the stoma. Stoma prolapse may be managed by conservative or surgical intervention. Surgical intervention is required if there is bowel ischemia, bowel obstruction, or prolapse of excessive length and unreducible segment of bowel. Conservative management includes reducing the stoma while in a supine position to decrease the intraabdominal pressure, then applying continuous gentle pressure at the distal portion of the prolapse until the stoma returns to skin level.

Retraction of the stoma below skin level can occur in the early postoperative period due to tension on the bowel or mesentery or related to breakdown at the mucocutaneous junction. Late retraction usually occurs as a result of tension on the bowel from abdominal distention, most likely as a result of intraperitoneal tumor growth or ascites. Stomal retraction is managed by modification of the pouching system—for example, by using a convex appliance to accommodate changes in skin contour. Stomas that retract below the fascia level require prompt surgical intervention.

Stenosis of the stoma can occur at the skin level or at the level of the fascia. Stenosis that interferes with normal bowel elimination requires intervention.

Peristomal Skin Problems

Peristomal skin complications commonly include mechanical breakdown, chemical breakdown, rash, and allergic reaction. Mechanical breakdown is caused by trauma to the epidermal skin layer. This is most often related to frequent appliance changes that cause shearing or tearing to the epidermal skin. The result is denuded skin or erythematous, raw, moist, and painful skin. The use of pectin-based powder with or without a light coating of skin sealant aids in healing and protecting the skin from further damage, while allowing appliance adherence.

Chemical breakdown is caused by prolonged contact of urine or fecal effluent with the peristomal skin. Inappropriate use of adhesive skin solvents may also result in skin breakdown. The result of chemical breakdown is denudation of the peristomal skin that has been exposed to the caustic effects of the stool, urine, or adhesive solvents. Prompt recognition and management are essential. Modification of the pouching system, such as using a convex wafer instead of a flat wafer or adding protective skin products such as a paste (or both), can be used to correct the underlying problem. Instructing patients and caregivers to thoroughly cleanse the skin with plain water after using the skin solvent can eliminate the problem of denuded skin.

A peristomal fungal rash can occur as a result of excessive moisture or antibiotic administration that results in overgrowth of yeast in the bowel or, at the skin level, as a result of perspiration under a pouch or leakage of urine or stool under the barrier. The rash is characterized as having a macular, red border with a moist, red to yellow center; it is usually pruritic. Application of antifungal powder, such as nystatin powder, to the affected areas usually produces a prompt response. Blotting the powder with skin preparation or sealant may allow the pouching system to adhere more effectively.

Allergic reactions are most often caused by the barrier and tape used for the pouching system. Erythematous vesicles and pruritus characterize the area involved. Management includes removal of the offending agent.

Principles and Products for Pouching a Stoma

The continuous outflow of urine or stool from the stoma requires the individual to wear an external appliance at all times. Ideally, the stoma protrudes one-half to three-fourths of an inch above the skin surface, to allow the urine or stool to drain efficiently into a pouch. The objectives of stoma management are to protect the peristomal skin, contain output, and control odor.

The skin around the stoma should be cleaned and thoroughly dried before the appliance is positioned over the stoma. An effective pouch should adhere for at least 3 days, although this is not always possible. If no leakage occurs, the same pouch may remain adhered to the skin for up to 10 days. It should then be changed for hygienic reasons and to observe the peristomal area. Today, there is an ever-changing supply of new appliances. Materials and design are being updated rapidly to provide the consumer with the best protection and easiest care. Factors to consider when choosing a pouch include the consistency and type of effluent, the contour of the abdomen, the size and shape of the stoma, and the extent of protrusion, as well as patient preferences.

Skin barriers, skin sealants, powders such as Stomahesive powder or karaya powder, and pastes such as Stomahesive paste or karaya paste are available to protect the peristomal skin from the caustic effects of urine or stool. These products may also be used to aid in the healing of peristomal skin problems.

Belts and binders are available to assist in maintaining pouch adherence and for management of certain stoma problems. Table 7.3 presents an overview of pouching options for patients with fecal or urinary diversions.

Interventions

Prevention of Complications

Stoma surgery performed as a palliative measure is not intended to provide a cure but, rather, to alleviate difficulties such as obstruction, pain, or severe incontinence. Unfortunately, at a difficult time in patients' and families' lives, the created stoma disrupts normal physical appearance, normal elimination of urine or stool, and control of elimination with, in some cases, loss of body parts and/or sexual function. The patient then has to learn to care for the

Table 7.3 Pouch Options		
Type	**Barrier**	**Odor-Proof Pouch**
One-piece	Flat	Open end with clip (ileostomy with colostomy)
Two-piece	Convex	Closed end (colostomy)
	Cut-to-fit precut	Spout opening (urostomy)

stoma or allow someone else to care for them. Physically and psychologically, the patient has to come to terms with the presence of the stoma, its function, and care. This takes time and energy to cope emotionally, physically, and socially.

Educating the patient and family regarding management issues related to ostomy care and palliation could assist in the physical and psychological adaptation to the ostomy. Additional therapies that may be required for treatment of the underlying disease or a new disease process, such as progressed or recurrent cancer, may affect the activity of the stoma or the peristomal skin.

Management

Controlling odor, reducing gas, and preventing or managing diarrhea or constipation are management issues related to patients with a colostomy.

Odor can be controlled by ensuring that the pouch seal is tight, that odor-proof pouches are used, and that a clean pouch opening is maintained. In addition, deodorants such as bismuth subgallate or chlorophyllin copper complex may be taken orally. Gas can be reduced by decreasing intake of gas-producing foods such as broccoli, cabbage, beans, and beer. Peppermint or chamomile tea may be effective in gas reduction.

Diarrhea can be managed as in a patient with an intact rectum and anus. Diarrhea may be a result of viral illness or use of a chemotherapeutic agent. Management includes increased fluid intake, a low-fiber and low-fat diet, and administration of antidiarrhea medications such as loperamide (Imodium), bismuth subsalicylate (Pepto-Bismol), or diphenoxylate plus atropine (Lomotil) by prescription. If the patient irrigates, it is necessary to hold irrigation until formed stools return.

Constipation more commonly occurs in patients with advanced malignancies due to the affects of analgesic use, reduced activity level, and reduced dietary fiber intake. Management of constipation includes administration of laxatives such as milk of magnesia, mineral oil, or lactulose and initiation of a plan for prevention of constipation with use of stool softeners and laxatives as needed. Cleansing irrigation may be necessary for patients who normally do not irrigate. Cleansing irrigation is performed as described previously for individuals with a colostomy who irrigate for control of bowel movements.

Skin protection, fluid and electrolyte maintenance, prevention of blockage, and modification of medications are management issues related to an ileostomy.

Leakage of effluent can cause chemical skin breakdown and pain from the irritated skin. The ET nurse can work with the patient and family to determine the cause of the effluent leak. It may be necessary to modify the pouching system, to ensure a proper fit. The peristomal skin may need to be treated with a powder or skin sealant, or both, to aid in healing.

The transit time of food and wastes through the gastrointestinal system and out through the ileostomy is rapid and potentially contributes to dehydration and fluid and electrolyte imbalance. Ensuring adequate fluid and electrolyte intake is essential and may be accomplished by ingestion of sports drinks or nutrition shakes. Patients with an ileostomy are instructed to include fiber in their diet, to bulk stools and promote absorption of nutrition and medications.

Food blockage occurs when undigested food particles or medications partially or completely obstruct the stoma outlet at the fascia level. It is necessary to instruct the patient and family about the signs of a blockage, including malodorous, high-volume liquid output or no output accompanied by abdominal cramping, distention, and/or nausea and vomiting. These symptoms should be reported as soon as they occur. Blockage is resolved by lavage or mini-irrigation performed by the physician or ET nurse. A catheter is gently inserted into the stoma until the blockage is reached, 30 to 60 mL of normal saline is instilled, and the catheter is removed to allow for the return. This process is repeated until the blockage has resolved. Patient teaching should be reinforced regarding the need to chew food well before swallowing, to prevent food blockage. Time-release tablets and enteric-coated medications should be avoided because of inadequate or unpredictable absorption. Medications often come in various forms, including liquid, noncoated, patch, rectal suppository, and subcutaneous or intravenous administration. Choosing the most appropriate route that provides the greatest efficacy for the individual is essential. For example, a transdermal patch may be used for analgesia instead of a time-released pain tablet. For patients who have an intact rectum that is no longer in continuity with the proximal bowel, rectal administration of medications is effective.

Management issues for an individual with an ileoconduit include prevention of a urinary tract infection, stone formation, peristomal skin protection, and odor control.

Each of these issues is preventable by the maintenance of dilute and acidic urine through adequate fluid intake (1800 to 2400 mL/day). Vitamin C (500 to 1000 mg/day) and citrus fruits and drinks may assist in accomplishing acidic urine.

Alkaline urine can cause encrustations on the stoma and peristomal skin damage with prolonged exposure. Acetic acid soaks may be applied three or four times per day to treat the encrustations until they dissolve.

Adjustments in the pouching system may be necessary to prevent leakage of urine onto the skin, and the temporary addition of powder, paste, skin sealant, or some combination of these products may be needed to aid healing of the affected skin.

Conclusion

Skin disorders are both emotionally and physically challenging for patients and caregivers. Cutaneous symptoms may be the result of disease progression (e.g., malignant wounds, fistula development), complications associated with end-stage disease or the end of life (e.g., pressure ulcers), or simple changes in function of urinary or fecal diversions. All cutaneous symptoms require attention to basic care issues, creativity in management strategies, and thoughtful attention to the psychosocial implications of cutaneous manifestations. Palliative care intervention strategies for skin disorders reflect an approach similar to those for nonpalliative care. Although the goals of care do not include curing the condition, they always include alleviating the distressing symptoms and improving quality of life. The most distressing symptoms associated with skin disorders are odor, exudate, and pain. The importance of attention to skin disorders for palliative care is related to the major effect of these conditions on the quality of life and general psychological well-being of the patient.

References

1. Nashan D, Meiss F, Braun-Falco M, Reichenberger S. Cutaneous metastases from internal malignancies. *Dermatol Ther.* 2010;*23*:567–580.

2. Alcarez I, Cerroni L, Rütten A, et al. Cutaneous metastases from internal malignancies: a clinicopathologic and immunohistochemical review. *Am J Dermatopathol.* 2012;*34*:347–393.

3. Bergstrom KJ. Assessment and management of fungating wounds. *J WOCN.* 2011;*38*:31–37.

4. Nashan D, Müller ML, Braun-Falco M, et al. Cutaneous metastasis of visceral tumors: a review. *J Cancer Res Clin Oncol.* 2009;*135*:1–14.

5. Grocott P, Gethin G, Probst S. Malignant wound management in advanced illness: new insights. *Curr Opin Support Palliat Care.* 2013;*7*:101–105.

6. Chrisman CA. Care of chronic wounds in palliative care and end-of-life patients. *Int Wound J.* 2010;*7*:214–235.

7. Wilkins RG, Unverdorben M. Wound cleaning and wound healing: a concise review. *Adv Skin Wound Care.* 2013;*26*:160–163.

8. Powers JG, Morton LM, Phillips TJ. Dressings for chronic wounds. *Dermatol Ther.* 2013;*26*:197–206.

9. da Costa Santos CM, de Mattos Pimenta CA, Nobre MR. A systematic review of topical treatments to control the odor of malignant fungating wounds. *J Pain Symptom Manage.* 2010;*39*(6):1065–1076.

10. Storm-Versloot MN, Vos CG, Ubbink DT, Vermeulen H. Topical silver for preventing wound infection. *Cochrane Database Syst Rev.* 2010;(3):CD006478.

11. Recka K, Montagnini M, Vitale CA. Management of bleeding associated with malignant wounds. *J Palliat Med.* 2012;*15*:952–954.

12. Parley P. Should topical opioid analgesics be regarded as effective and safe when applied to chronic cutaneous lesions? *J Pharm Pharmacol.* 2011;*63*:747–756.

13. LeBon B, Zeppetella G, Higginson IJ. Effectiveness of topical administration of opioids in palliative care: a systematic review. *J Pain Symptom Manage.* 2009;*37*:913–917.

14. Wiltshire BL. Challenging enterocutaneous fistula: a case presentation. *J Wound Ostomy Cont Nurs.* 1996;*23*:297–301.

15. Wainstein DE, Fernandez E, Gonzalez D, et al. Treatment of high-output enterocutaneous fistulas with a vacuum-compaction device: a ten-year experience. *World J Surg.* 2008;*32*(3):430–435.

Chapter 8

Pruritus, Fever, and Sweats

Philip J. Larkin

Pruritus

Introduction

Pruritus has been defined as "an unpleasant sensation that elicits either a conscious or reflex desire to scratch." A recent Cochrane systematic review of pruritus in palliative care patients describes it as a pathologic condition exhibited by an intense sensation of itch that triggers scratching to alleviate discomfort.[1] It is seen across both malignant and nonmalignant disease, notably in hematologic cancers, cancers of the biliary tract, and hepatic and uremic disease.[2,3] Pruritus remains poorly defined and understood, particularly within a palliative care context. Pruritus should not be considered simply a skin disorder, but rather a systemic problem for which there are multiple causes. Four descriptive categories have been noted that highlight the challenge in diagnosis and management:

- Prurioreceptive (within the skin)
- Neuropathic (damage to the afferent pathway)
- Neurogenic (cerebrally induced)
- Psychogenic (related to psychiatric disorder)

As in many palliative care clinical situations, it is difficult to isolate these entirely, and some degree of overlap is likely. Why scratching relieves an itch is not fully understood; there would appear to be some physiologic synchronicity between pruritus and pain, given the fact that similar chemical messengers excite the unmyelinated C fibers. It may be that a specific subset of these fibers responds particularly to pruritus-inducing stimuli and mediators such as histamine and prostaglandins. The ability to trace the neurologic pathways of histamine through the dorsal horn and into the thalamus and sensorimotor cortex would appear to confirm this as the primary mediator of itch.[4] However, other peripheral mediators have been identified, including serotonin, prostaglandin, and dopamine.[4]

Sleep deprivation and broken skin from scratching are noted phenomena, and the impact of chronic unrelieved pruritus has been equated to the debilitation associated with chronic pain. Its subjective nature makes it both unrelenting and unpredictable, and although scratching behavior is observable and measurable, the burden experienced by the patient is not conducive to measurement.

Nursing Assessment and Differential Diagnosis

In considering the categories of pruritus noted previously, it is important to remember that it may be both localized and generalized. There is a distinction between primary or idiopathic pruritus (for which no cause can be determined) and secondary pruritus (related to systemic or localized disease), and decisions about the extent of investigation of the systemic problem need to be considered. General skin disorders such as eczema, psoriasis, or infestation should be ruled out, or treated as necessary, before attributing the problem to an internal cause. However, systemic etiology may be present in up to 40% of all cases. Therefore, in cases of nonspecific generalized pruritus, it is important to monitor for the development of systemic disease over time. Table 8.1 lists some of the key causes of pruritus based on Bernhard's classification, with a specific focus on those causes seen in palliative care practice.

Specific questions that may form part of a clinical assessment include the following:

- Can a location for itch be specified?
- Is there presence or absence of rash?
- Is there evidence of a fungal or parasitic infection?
- Is there evidence of broken or dry skin?
- Is there bleeding or seepage of serous fluid?

It is important to quantify the level of discomfort imposed by itch. A thorough clinical assessment is imperative, including a review of medications, particularly new use of opioids. The patient should also be questioned sensitively about his or her personal hygiene regimen and use of specific deodorants, lotions, and bath products. Associations with food, weather, and exposure to new environments (e.g., pets, new bedding or clothes) should also be explored. If appropriate in the context of palliative stage of disease, laboratory blood tests may be useful in diagnosis. A complete blood count, including urea and creatinine, should be considered, as well as tests to rule out endocrine or metabolic dysfunction (e.g., serum glucose, thyroxine, and bilirubin levels).

Medical Management

Owing to the breadth of possible causes for pruritus, management needs to balance the response between intervention, patient perception of the problem, and clinical status. Centrally acting antihistamine preparations can be effective but sedating and are therefore best administered at night. Because the symptom may be exacerbated at night, the sedative effect may not be a problem and might even assist the patient in getting to sleep. However, in terms of life quality, oversedation would not be an appropriate palliative care response and thus would need careful monitoring, and the evidence for the use of antihistamine preparations is limited.[4]

A wide array of medications have been efficacious in the treatment of pruritus. Particularly when pruritus is considered opioid induced and not responsive to antihistamine therapy, rifampicin has been shown to achieve a rapid resolution of the symptom.

Table 8.1 Key Causes of Pruritus

Bernhard's Classification	Overall Problem	Clinical Presentation
Dermatologic	Generalized skin problems	Psoriasis, eczema, urticaria, scabies, pediculosis, xerosis (dry skin)
		Contact dermatitis, atopic dermatitis, allergy (e.g., nickel, bathing products)
	Medication (including hypersensitivity)	Opioids, amphetamines, acetylsalicylic acid, quinidine
	Blood dyscrasias (including hematologic malignancy)	Iron deficiency anemia
		Polycythemia rubra vera
		Leukemias
		Lymphomas
		Hodgkin's disease
Systemic	Organ failure	Liver failure (malignant cholestasis, primary biliary cirrhosis, hepatitis)
		Renal failure (uremia, postdialysis dermatosis)
	Endocrine and metabolic dysfunction	Diabetes mellitus
		Hyperthyroidism/ hypothyroidism
		Hyperparathyroidism/ hypoparathyroidism
		Zinc deficiency
	Connective tissue disorder	Systemic lupus erythematosus
		Chronic graft versus host disease
Neuropathic/neurogenic (including neuroanatomic and neurochemical disorders)	Chronic and potentially life-limiting disease	Neuroendocrine tumors
		Paraneoplastic tumors
		Multiple sclerosis
		Stroke
		Brain injury
		Post–herpes zoster infection
		Syphilis

Another medication that has been demonstrated as beneficial in the treatment of pruritus is ondansetron, commonly used in the treatment of chemotherapy-induced nausea and vomiting. As a 5-HT3 serotonin antagonist, ondansetron has shown a dramatic effect in reducing itch following intravenous infusion and regular oral administration in patients with malignant cholestasis and has also been noted as effective in other patient populations. Other potential choices of treatment would include topical treatments, local anesthetics, and antidepressants such as mirtazapine, which has antiserotogenic effects at the 5-HT2 and 5-HT3 receptors and offers benefits similar to those of ondansetron. Gabapentin has also been used to good effect, as has buprenorphine, with a very low dose of naloxone in combination to manage brachioradial pruritus.

Topical and systemic corticosteroids have a place in treatment, although their use may be limited because of potential side effects. Paroxetine has also been considered most effective with stronger supporting evidence for its use.[1] However, it is important to note that most of the evidence available on the treatment of pruritus is limited to clinical reports, case histories, and small-scale studies. In the palliative context, particularly when there may be multi-organ failure, systemic treatment choices may be very limited, especially if opiate use for optimal pain control is not stabilized. Therefore, a program of nursing management is an essential component of the approach to care.

Nursing Management

Regardless of cause, the patient complaint focuses on the skin, and nursing management should endeavor to provide the highest standard of skin care to supplement medical intervention. Although topical treatment alone may have minimal benefit, it may contribute to relieving the patient's discomfort. Skin cleansing is important, along with the prevention of xerosis (dry skin), which may exacerbate the pruritus. Bathing may assist hydration in the short term, but the essential need is to keep the skin moist. Emollient oils should be added to the bath near the end because doing so at the beginning may have a drying effect. A "soak and seal" method that involves bathing, patting (not rubbing) the skin dry and then adding a moisturizer may be beneficial. The choice of skin cleanser and moisturizer should ideally be pH neutral and free from fragrance and alcohol. Soap and talcum powder should be avoided owing to their drying properties. The water content of the product should be relatively low because it may evaporate quickly.

Frequent application of moisturizer and the use of soft, cool clothing, preferably cotton, should be encouraged. Topical antihistamine preparations, such as an oil-based calamine lotion, may soothe excoriated and scratched skin. Cool packs, cool oatmeal baths, and loose, light bedding can be beneficial, particularly when settling the patient for sleep. An ambient room temperature (cooler rather than warmer) may be relaxing, although this is less easy to regulate when the patient is hospitalized. The patient should be advised to keep nails short and to rub or pat rather than scratch, if at all possible. A physical examination for damage to skin or evidence of a secondary infection should be carried out regularly and any damage or infection treated accordingly.

Fever

Introduction

Fever is defined as a rise in body temperature exceeding 38° C (100.4° F) from the norm (37°± 1° C) (98.78° F).[5] Table 8.2 outlines the many and varied causes of fever, most of which have direct relevance for palliative care patients. Notably, patients with advanced dementia may have fever as a common symptom of their end-of-life stage of illness.[6] Further, older people may exhibit an altered febrile response, which makes the assessment of body temperature a limited diagnostic tool. The particular problems of fever in hematologic conditions as part of a spectrum of symptoms (fever, infection, anemia, and bleeding) has prompted a call for greater integration with palliative care services.

The presentation of fever often manifests in three stages. These have been described as chill, fever, and flush:

1. *Chill phase:* The body attempts to respond to the raised thermal set point by vasoconstriction of the skin to prevent heat loss and muscle contraction to generate heat. This results in shivering and, in marked cases, rigors.

2. *Fever:* The second phase is dominated by a sensation of warmth, flushed skin, lethargy, weakness, and possibly dehydration, delirium, and/or seizure. This occurs as the core body temperature rises to the new set point. During fever, the basal metabolic rate is increased to meet new tissue and oxygenation requirements by up to 13% per 1° C increase.

3. *Flush:* In the third and final phase, the core temperature attempts to normalize with the new set point through vasodilation and sweating (diaphoresis).

Table 8.2 Key Causes of Fever

Causative Factors	Causative Agent
Infection	Bacteria, fungi, viruses, parasites, tuberculosis, hepatitis, endocarditis, contaminated food.
Inflammation	Trauma, surgery, splenectomy heat, ulcerative colitis, pulmonary embolism, radiation, gastrointestinal bleeding.
Cancer treatment	Chemotherapeutic agents, blood products, immunosuppression, neutropenia, external devices for venous access, catheters
Tumors	Hodgkin's and non-Hodgkin's lymphoma; leukemia; carcinoma of the liver, lung, and genitourinary systems; adrenal cancer; Ewing's sarcoma; renal disease; tumors affecting the thermoregulatory system of the brain
Autoimmune disease	Rheumatoid arthritis, connective tissue disorder, anaphylaxis, polymyalgia
Neurologic disorder	Spinal or brain injury or infection, stroke
Environmental	Allergens
Other	Constipation, dehydration, medication

For the palliative care population, particularly patients with a cancer diagnosis, episodes of neutropenia, infection, and fever are not uncommon. As the patient becomes increasingly immunosuppressed, attack by pyrogens may lead to overwhelming sepsis and death if left untreated. Recent review of approaches to febrile neutropenia would argue that risk stratification tools such as the Multinational Association for Supportive Care in Cancer Index (assessing high or low complication risk to determine treatment options) should be used.[5] Although there are challenges in terms of the sensitivity of risk stratification tools, there is evidence that outpatient treatment, even with intravenous therapy and early discharge in cases of hospitalization, leads to higher health outcomes. As always in palliative care, the justification for aggressive intervention needs to be considered in relation to the patient's overall health status.

The use of blood transfusions in palliative care is a debate in itself, but the risk for hemolytic reaction and associated fever is possible. Therefore, for many reasons, its benefit should be carefully evaluated. Given that bacterial infection can account for up to 90% of fevers, anything that might introduce infection through damaged skin integrity (such as venous access and urinary catheters) also warrants judicious use and scrupulous aseptic practice. Medications may also trigger a febrile response, most commonly penicillins, cephalosporins, antifungals (e.g. amphotericin), and, of course, chemotherapy agents (e.g., bleomycin). Pneumocystis *jiroveci* pneumonia, commonly associated with HIV/AIDS, is increasingly prevalent in non-HIV-positive populations and often overlooked in terms of a causative factor, even though it has a noted prevalence in the cancer population.

Nursing Assessment and Differential Diagnosis

The differential diagnosis of fever will determine realistic goals and the most appropriate plan of care. Clearly, a thorough physical examination and recent history are essential.[7] Questions to consider during the assessment include the following:

- Is there evidence suggestive of a respiratory tract infection?
- Is there evidence suggestive of a urinary infection?
- How long has the patient been febrile?
- What is the pattern of the fever (day or night, number of peaks of temperature over 24 hours)?
- What medication or treatment is in progress or recently completed?
- Has there been a recent blood transfusion?
- Have there been any recent invasive procedures?
- Have blood tests been obtained?
- Is there evidence of damage to the skin integument?
- Are there any venous access devices or catheters?

Medical Management

In the palliative context, the degree to which fever is treated aggressively raises the debate about burden over benefit—life quality versus the risk for prolonged dying. The complexity of the decision whether to use antibiotics is evidenced by the diversity of opinion within the literature as to their value and efficacy. Whatever decision is made regarding antibiotics, it is important that a plan of care includes decisions on the conditions that would herald cessation of treatment.

Acetaminophen has the benefit of offering relatively rapid response to pyrexia and is available in a variety of forms—tablet, suspension, suppository, or intravenous (although the expense may complicate use). Aspirin, if tolerated, may also be effective. Corticosteroids also hold antipyretic properties, although their benefit needs to be weighed against the possible side effects. Antipyretic medication should be administered regularly and not on an as-needed basis, or it may induce fluctuating patterns of fever and sweating. More intensive management may be required, depending on the cause of the fever. Fever related to tumor may be responsive to radiation, if the patient's condition is stable enough for treatment. Further, neuroleptic agents such as chlorpromazine may be beneficial when the fever is centrally mediated.

Nursing Management

Comfort should be the key priority in the palliative approach. It is important to obtain a balance between "cooling" and "cold," the latter of which may only exacerbate the discomfort caused by shivering and heat generation.

Bathing with tepid water, drying off gently, and using light bedding may add to comfort, but cold packs and ice should be avoided.

Cool fluids should be encouraged, and attention to mouth and skin care is imperative, particularly in cases in which there is a risk for dehydration.

A fan should be used to cool the ambient air and not be focused directly on the patient.

Sweats and Hot Flashes

Introduction

Although sweats are considered one of the major problems experienced by patients, research evidence for the management and treatment of sweats remains sparse. Night sweats have been identified as a significant problem for advanced cancer patients, with a prevalence of up to 48%. Age, gender, ambient temperature, and exercise are all known to influence the amount of sweating that takes place. Table 8.3 lists common causes of sweating.

Hot flashes are reported in up to 75% of menopausal women and described as a sensation of heat, associated with flushing, palpitations, and anxiety.[8] Completely unpredictable, hot flashes interfere greatly with life quality and, in particular, sleep. They are common in patients with breast cancer because of estrogen deprivation and are noted in up to 70% of breast cancer patients on tamoxifen therapy. The problem is also seen in men with prostate cancer.

Beyond breast and prostate cancer, sweating is noted in a variety of illnesses, including malignancy. Hyperhidrosis (excessive sweating) may be directly related to disease or may have no evident cause. In each case, it can be localized or generalized and may present as "night sweats," as described at the start of this section.

Table 8.3 Key Causes of Sweating and Hot Flashes	
Disorder	Examples
Endocrine disorders	Estrogen deficiency, hyperthyroidism, hypoglycemia
Malignancy	Lymphoma, breast cancer, prostate cancer, neuroendocrine tumors
Chronic infection	Tuberculosis, lupus
Medication (including withdrawal from)	Opioids, barbiturates, estrogen depriving agents (e.g., tamoxifen)
Emotion	Stress, anxiety, fear

Nursing Assessment and Differential Diagnosis

Key assessment questions that may be helpful when ascertaining the impact of the problem on the life quality of the patient include the following:

- How often do you find yourself sweating?
- How would you describe these sweats?
- Are they a particular problem at night?
- Do you have any other problems when you sweat, such as nausea, vomiting, or feeling faint, anxious, or fearful?
- Have you changed any medication recently?
- Is your sweating all over your body or confined to certain parts?
- Have you identified anything that seems to make your sweating better or worse?
- How much of a problem is this sweating for you?

Medical Management

Unfortunately, drug therapy options for the management of sweating are relatively limited, and there is very little evidence beyond case reports and pilot trials to support the use of any specific treatment. Medications that work as antispasmodics and anticholinergics have also demonstrated some benefit. One option is the use of thioridazine, a phenothiazine, antipsychotic, and antimuscarinic agent.[9] A further small-scale study has indicated benefit with the use of the cannabinoid nabilone for persistent night sweats.

There is a growing body of research looking at options for the management of hot flashes and a number of small studies in relation to the use of progestational agents (e.g., megestrol acetate), clonidine, selective serotonin reuptake inhibitors, and gabapentin have been proposed.[9,10] However, there is contrasting evidence in relation to the use and efficacy of hormone replacement therapy (HRT), which is a standard treatment offered to healthy menopausal women; therefore, in addition to the progestational agents, HRT is not recommended for women with a history of breast cancer.

Given the link to "menopausal" symptoms, a number of nonpharmacologic preparations have been proposed, including evening primrose oil, phytoestrogens, and herbs. Although there is weak evidence for the use of complementary and supportive therapies, there is some suggestion that relaxation techniques to address the emotional component of the symptom may be beneficial.[8] Cognitive behavioral therapy and yoga may also be of benefit. However, the evidence remains weak, and the discomfort associated with this symptom indicates the need for sensitive and responsive nursing care.

Nursing Management

It is argued that the ethics of care begin with that which is most basic, and the care for the body is an example of that basic—but notably not simple—care. Because the burden of sweats on the patient's quality of life would appear to be great, nursing care must include an approach that addresses the immediate discomfort and anxiety. Patients should be advised to have extra changes of nightwear (or day clothes if the symptoms are not restricted to the night) and additional bedding available. Just as in the fever-type response, the patient may feel cold following diaphoresis and so should be kept comfortable in an ambient temperature while washing and changing. Similar to the treatment of fever, cool (but not cold) fluids should be encouraged to avoid dehydration because the risk for multiple sweats in one night is not uncommon. Avoiding hot and spicy foods and wearing loose clothing may also assist in maintaining comfort.

Patients may fear that their sweating indicates a deterioration or recurrence of disease. Night sweats may indicate this in the case of lymphoma. The patient may be embarrassed by the symptom and withdraw from social events. Gentle discussion about the problem and reassurance that efforts are being made to find a solution may ease distress. Careful observation of factors relating to the sweats (time, duration, extent, patient response) may indicate a possible treatment pathway. Referral for complementary and supportive therapy should always be considered for the practical and emotional benefit it can bring.

Conclusion

Perhaps of all symptoms that palliative care patients endure, those of pruritus, fever, and sweats most remind nurses of their fundamental grounding in caring for others. The care given to patients with these symptoms is reflective of skills learned and nurtured throughout the nursing career, and then specifically honed to meet end-of-life needs. Comfort remains the key priority, particularly when drug therapy may have limited effect. The "benefit–burden calculus" should be uppermost in the mind with respect to the goals of treatment. As the clinical team members with closest proximity to the patient, nurses may need to voice their concerns, and the concerns of others, when an intervention appears to be unwarranted or even futile.

The attention to detail required in order to address these symptoms highlights the importance to palliative nursing of those philosophical constructs noted at the beginning of this chapter—hope, dignity, comfort, and empathy.

References

1. Xander C, Meerpohl JJ, Galandi D, et al. Pharmacological interventions for pruritus in adult palliative care patients. *Cochrane Database Syst Rev.* 2013(6):CD008320.

2. Chaing HC, Huang V, Cornelius LA. Cancer and itch. *Semin Cutaneous Med Surg.* 2011;30(2):107–112.

3. Metz M, Ständer S. Chronic pruritus: pathogenesis, clinical aspects and treatment. *J Eur Acad Dermatol Venerol.* 2010;24:1249–1260.

4. Yosipovitch G, Barnard JD. Chronic pruritus. *N Engl J Med.* 2013;368:1625–1634.

5. de Naurois J, Novitzky-Basso I, Gill MJ, et al. Management of febrile neutropenia: ESMO clinical practice guidelines. *Ann Oncol.* 2010;21(Suppl 5):v252–v256.

6. Pascoe J. Developments in the management of febrile neutropaenia. *Br J Cancer.* 2011;105:597–598.

7. Dalal S, Zhukovsky DS. Pathophysiology and management of fever. *J Support Oncol.* 2006;4:9–16.

8. Morrow PKH, Mattair DN, Hortobagyi GN. Hot flashes: a review of pathophysiology and treatment modalities. *Oncologist.* 2011;16:1658–1664.

9. Loprinzi CL, Barton DL, Sloan JA, et al. Mayo Clinic and North Central Cancer Treatment Group hot flash studies: a 20-year experience. *Menopause.* 2008;15:655–660.

10. Bordeleau L, Pritchard KI, Loprinzi CL, et al. Multicenter, randomized, cross-over clinical trial of venlafaxine versus gabapentin for the management of hot flashes in breast cancer survivors. *J Clin Oncol.* 2010;28:5147–5152.

Chapter 9

Neurologic Disorders

Margaret A. Schwartz

Introduction

The palliative care nurse is likely to encounter a patient with an advanced neurologic disorder or a medical condition with neurologic complications and therefore should be prepared for the variety of symptoms and diagnoses that are associated with neurologic diseases. This chapter addresses broad symptom categories as well as common neurologic diseases with heavy symptom burden deserving of special attention.

Abnormal Movements

The human body is capable of a broad variety of involuntary and abnormal movements—shivering, tremor, seizures, fasciculations, myoclonus, and chorea to name a few. Table 9.1 provides definitions of the abnormal movements most frequently encountered.

Seizures

Seizures are defined as electrical discharges of the cerebral cortex with resulting changes in the functions of the central nervous system (CNS).[1] Any condition that disturbs the normal environment of the CNS can result in a seizure. There are a number of conditions that increase the risk for an epileptic event. The most common of these include acute metabolic derangements, medications and substances, space-occupying lesions of the brain, ischemic events, and infection (Table 9.2). It is important to note that a single seizure does not constitute epilepsy.

Witnessing a seizure can be a traumatic event for caregivers and providers. Additionally, the emotional burden for patients with seizures is great:

- Impaired sleep
- Mood disorders
- Pain
- Psychological distress

Seizure definitions are included in Table 9.3. Unchecked, seizures can result in significant morbidity—delirium, physical injury, aspiration, rhabdomyolysis and renal injury, pain, temporary paralysis, and loss of function. Among oncology patients, there are a number of factors increasing the risk for

Table 9.1 Commonly Encountered Neurologic Definitions

Agraphia	Inability to write. Of note, agraphia rarely occurs in isolation.
Akathisia	A sensation of restlessness, often accompanied by a compulsion to move the effected limbs. Most commonly found in patients with Parkinson's disease, dementia, and those receiving neuroleptics.
Alexia	Inability to read.
Aphasia	Impaired verbal or written communication because of an acquired insult to the brain. *Expressive aphasia* is an impairment in the ability to generate spoken language (also known as anterior/nonfluent/Broca's/motor aphasia). *Receptive aphasia* is difficulty or inability to understand spoken word (also known as posterior/fluent/Wernicke's/sensory aphasia). Global aphasia is the inability to use language. Patients with global aphasia can neither read nor write.
Asterixis	Also known as "flapping tremor," asterixis is commonly encountered in patients with metabolic and toxic encephalopathy (most notably in ammonia retention). It is characterized by irregular lapses of a sustained posture, often followed by an overcorrection. It is also observed in neck and arms of the drowsy person.
Ataxia	Lack of coordination of voluntary movements.
Athetosis	Involuntary and abnormal slow, complex writhing movements. Most commonly involves fingers, hands, toes, and feet. Encountered in various forms with encephalitis, hepatic encephalopathy, Parkinson's disease, Huntington's disease, and cerebral palsy.
Chorea	Arrhythmic movements characterized by a writhing, rapid, and jerky quality. The movements are purposeless and involuntary. Often accompanied by a general state of hypotonia—the limbs hang slack. The major distinguishing feature of Huntington's disease.
Clonus	Rhythmic contraction and relaxation of antagonistic muscle groups.
Corticospinal tracts	The neurons connecting the cortex of the brain (gray matter) with the lower motor neurons in the ventral horn of the spinal cord.
Dysarthria	Impaired speech output due to oral, lingual, or pharyngeal motor impairment.
Dyskinesia	A wide-encompassing term meaning abnormal movement. Movements can be intermittent or persistent. In tardive dyskinesia, the movements are slow, rhythmic, and automatic.
Dysmetria	Ataxia with overshoot or undershoot of movement, dysmetria results from difficulty processing or perceiving the position of the body in relation to its surroundings.
Dysphagia	Impaired ability to swallow in a coordinated and timely fashion.
Dystonia	A unilateral movement defined by involuntary muscle contraction of both the agonist and antagonist muscles. The result is the limb held in a twisted, distorted posture. Can affect a limb, the head and neck, the face, or the spinal muscles.

(continued)

Table 9.1 (Continued)

Fasciculation	A small, localized pattern of muscle contraction and relaxation, often observable through the skin. Commonly noted in the eyelid of healthy individuals, it can also be seen in ALS, progressive spinal muscle atrophy, or states causing nerve fiber irritability (dehydration, muscular exhaustion, metabolic imbalance).
Lower motor neuron	The neurons that connect the upper motor neurons to the muscle fibers. Lower motor neurons originate in the ventral horn of the spinal cord or in the brainstem motor nerve nuclei and terminate on the neuromuscular plate of effector muscles.
Myoclonus	Rapid and irregular shocklike contractions of a group of muscles. The most commonly experienced myoclonic events are hiccups and "sleep starts." Palliative care nurses are likely to encounter opioid-induced myoclonus.
Myokymia	The irregular firing of several motor units, seen as a rippling of the skin.
Nystagmus	Involuntary jerking movement of the eyes in either a lateral or vertical direction.
Opsoclonus	Involuntary and irregular multidirectional movement of the eyes.
Seizures	Aberrant electrical activity of a part or the entire cortex of the brain, resulting in altered neurologic functions.
Tardive dyskinesia	A specific dyskinesia characterized by repetitive and stereotyped movements, often of the face, mouth, and tongue. It is most commonly an effect of antipsychotic medications.
Tremor	Rhythmic contraction of a muscle or group of muscles in opposing directions.
Upper motor neuron	The motor neurons originating in the motor cortex of the brain or brainstem and carrying synapses down to the lower motor neurons. Upper motor neurons do not directly contact the target muscle.

seizures. Brain metastases, chemotherapy and radiation, and metabolic and endocrinologic changes in the patient with cancer increase the risk for seizures. In patients with primary brain tumors, the burden of seizures is staggering. There are many interventions available to the palliative care nurse to reduce the impact of seizures.

The palliative care nurse begins with a careful history and physical examination, including several key areas:

- Any new physical findings that may suggest an underlying physiologic change that has lowered the seizure threshold
- Review of recent medication changes
- Review of the history for substance abuse because patients newly abstinent from alcohol, benzodiazepines, opioids, or illicit substances are at elevated risk for seizures

When no source is immediately identified, radiographic or metabolic evaluation may be indicated if it is within the goals of care.

Family and patient teaching are important to dispel fear and to maximize patient comfort. Education goals focus on safety during seizures, post-ictal care, medications, eliminating the cause of the seizure when feasible, and when to contact the provider. Safety during a seizure focuses on minimizing

Table 9.2 Common Conditions Resulting in Seizures

Metabolic changes	Electrolyte imbalances
	Thyrotoxic storm
	Uremia
	Hypertensive encephalopathy
	Hypertension of pregnancy (eclampsia and preeclampsia)
	Fever
	Dehydration and overhydration
	Hyperventilation
Medication related, illicit substance related	Missed doses or withdrawal
	New medications
	Metabolite accumulation
Intracranial tumors	Metastatic tumors
	Primary central nervous system tumors
Ischemia	Stroke
	Diffuse cerebral hypoxia
Infections	Encephalitis
	Meningitis
	Intracranial abscess
	Parasitic lesions
Paraneoplastic syndromes	NMDA-receptor encephalitis
Trauma related	Motor vehicle crash
	Blow to head
	Explosion
Vascular lesions	Arteriovenous malformation
	Intracranial aneurysm
	Subdural hemorrhage or fluid collection
	Epidural hemorrhage
	Subarachnoid hemorrhage
Idiopathic or congenital disorders	Birth injury
	Congenital malformation
	Enzyme deficiencies
	Lysosomal storage disorders
	Channelopathies

injury—falls and physical trauma during clonic movements—as well as minimizing the length of seizure if possible. Padding the patient's surroundings (bed rails) is traditionally done for those with refractory seizures. See Box 9.1 for seizure first-aid and safety suggestions.

Placing objects in the mouth and restraining the patient are absolutely contraindicated. Patients should not be given food or liquid until they have fully recovered consciousness. Should the patient fail to regain full consciousness between seizures or continue to seize after several minutes—a condition known as status epilepticus—urgent action is required. Status epilepticus is treated as a serious and life-threatening situation requiring immediate administration of medication to break the seizures. If the seizure occurs in

Table 9.3 Seizure Definitions

Simple focal (partial) seizure	The uncontrolled electrical activity in a simple partial seizure is limited to a small area of the cortex. The resulting seizure is not accompanied by loss of consciousness. Symptoms include shaking of a single area of the body. Less commonly, simple partial seizures can result in abnormal sensations of the affected limb or in abnormal sensations such as auditory, visual, or gustatory changes. Rarely, simple partial seizures can result in behavior and emotional changes.
Complex focal (partial) seizure	Affecting a larger area of the brain, complex partial seizures result in impairments in the ability of the person to interact with his surroundings. Often starting with a blank look or staring spell and progressing to stereotyped, repetitive movements. Also termed *psychomotor seizures.*
Generalized seizure	The most common and obvious of the seizures. Generalized seizures involve the entire cortex of the brain. The typical generalized seizure begins with limb stiffening (tonic posturing) and a period of apnea or hypoventilation. This gives way to clonic movements (jerking of the limbs and/or head as muscles contract and relax together). During the clonic phase, breathing returns, although it is often irregular.
Absence seizure	A generalized seizure in which the patient abruptly ceases activity and stares blankly. The patient is unable to interact with the environment during the seizure. As soon as the seizure is finished, the patient returns to the activity preceding the ictal event.
Atonic seizure	Atonic (drop-attack/astatic/akinetic) seizures are generalized seizures resulting in an abrupt loss of postural tone. Loss of tone can vary from head drooping to full collapse.
Aura	In epilepsy, an aura is the initial phase of a focal seizure. It is generally experienced as a motor, sensory, autonomic, or psychic event. For some patients, the aura alone constitutes the seizure.
Epilepsy	A syndrome of repeated seizures.
Febrile seizure	A seizure occurring in infants and children (ages 6 months to 5 years) in the setting of a temperature usually above 38° C. Febrile seizures are usually a single generalized motor seizure as the patient's temperature peaks. Be certain to distinguish between febrile seizures and complicated febrile seizures, the latter occurring repeatedly during a febrile illness.
Ictal	Latin for "stroke," ictal has come to mean the height of a seizure or migraine.
Psychogenic nonepileptic seizures	Also called *pseudoseizures*, these are events characterized by changes in neurologic function in the absence of electroencephalographic changes indicating abnormal electrical activity of the cortex.
Status epilepticus	A cluster of seizures without return to full neurologic baseline between events or a single, ongoing seizure lasting more than a few minutes. Considered a medical emergency, status epilepticus carries an elevated risk for brain damage, hypoxia, and death.

the home, emergency medical services may be appropriate if consistent with the goals of care. Of note, there remain several states in the United States that require providers to report seizure events to the Department of Motor Vehicles. Certainly, patients with seizures should abstain from driving until cleared by a neurologist.

Of utmost importance for patient comfort and safety is to stop the seizure as it happens. Seizure-ablative medications may be limited by the specific

Box 9.1 Seizure Safety

Seizure First Aid

Prevent injury by moving furniture or hard objects out of the way.
Refrain from putting anything in the mouth of the patient.
Place a pillow or soft item under the patient's head.
Loosen tight clothing around the neck.

After-Seizure Care

Avoid situations dangerous to the epileptic patient (open flame, unaccompanied boating, swimming, tub-bathing)
Avoid seizure triggers (sleep deprivation, blood sugar lows, alcohol consumption, excess caffeine intake)

patient situation. The patient receiving hospice at home will likely be best served by administration of rapid-acting benzodiazepines. Orally administered concentrated lorazepam drops are readily available from the hospice pharmacy. Other choices include rectal diazepam gel, nasal lorazepam gel, or clonazepam wafers applied to the buccal surface. In the patient with intravenous access, slow intravenous push administration is generally the preferred choice.

Several issues require specific attention in the palliative care setting. In a patient with a reversible condition, antiepileptic drugs (AEDs) may not be required. Patients with epilepsy or significant risk for ongoing seizures will require careful consideration for AED choice. If the patient with metastatic or primary brain tumors has never experienced a seizure, the current recommendation is not to prophylactically administer anticonvulsants. For a brief overview of factors to be considered when introducing AEDs, see Box 9.2.

Box 9.2 Special Considerations When Introducing an Antiepileptic Drug

Drug interactions are common with antiepileptic drugs (AEDs), especially older-generation medications that induce the cytochrome P450 hepatic enzymes.
Many AEDs can alter mood and are used as psychotropic medications.
Carefully review comorbidities.
Phenytoin can cause osteoporosis, and topiramate can induce weight loss.
The patient with limited life expectancy, impaired level of consciousness, or diminished ability to swallow makes most oral AEDs a poor choice—consider scheduled benzodiazepines.
Most AEDs do not require drug level monitoring.
Dexamethasone is neither an antiepileptic medication nor a seizure-ablating drug.
Phenytoin increases metabolism of corticosteroids, and corticosteroids can alter the metabolism of phenytoin—consider a different AED.
Consultation with a neurologist may be warranted.

Notably, several choices have arisen in recent years for the patient with medically refractory seizures. A restrictive diet inducing a ketogenic state has been studied for decades for medically refractory childhood epilepsy with some success. Surgical options include resection of the seizure focus or lesion as well as vagal nerve stimulator placement. Careful consideration must be given to the life expectancy and appropriateness of the patient for such procedures and interventions.

Myoclonus

Myoclonus is a series of brief muscular contractions. The contractions are irregular in both the amplitude of contraction and rhythm and denote a disturbance of the CNS. There are a wide variety of myoclonic syndromes (see Table 9.4 for common causes of myoclonus).

The palliative care nurse begins with careful examination and review of medications. An interview of the patient and family may elicit a recent change. Renal impairment is associated with opioid-induced myoclonus (OIM). The patient or family will describe nonrhythmic jerking movements. Stimulation

Table 9.4 Causes of Myoclonus	
Drug related	Opioid-induced myoclonus
	Lithium toxicity
	Haloperidol
	Phenothiazines
	Cyclosporine
	β-Lactam antibiotics
	Antidepressants
Metabolic disorders	Hepatic encephalopathy
	Nicotinic acid deficiency
	Uremia
	Storage diseases
Inflammatory disorders	Thyroiditis
Infectious diseases	Whipple's disease of the central nervous system
	Tetanus
	Herpes zoster myelitis
Central nervous system disorders	Hypoxic brain injury
	Multiple sclerosis
	Paraneoplastic syndromes
	AIDS dementia complex
	Viral encephalitis
	Advanced dementias
	Cerebellar degenerative conditions
	Basal ganglia degenerative conditions
	Creutzfeldt-Jakob disease
	Parkinson's disease
	Subacute sclerosis panencephalitis
	Myoclonic epilepsy syndromes

of the patient or taping on the muscles may bring on or worsen myoclonus. Hyperalgesia and hallucinations in the setting of myoclonus raise the suspicion of OIM and should trigger an evaluation of pain medications.[2] The precise mechanisms behind OIM are unknown. The leading theorized mechanisms point to accumulation of neuroexcitatory metabolites, particularly hydromorphone-3-glucuronide and morphine-3-glucuronide, in the setting of impaired kidney function. Although higher doses of opioids are more commonly implicated in OIM, it can occur in patients with relatively low doses and preserved renal function. If OIM is suspected, opioid rotation, addition of a benzodiazepine such as clonazepam or midazolam, and a trial of adjuvant medications is indicated.[3,4]

In the patient with opsoclonus myoclonus syndrome, the myoclonus is typically diffuse or focal with titubation (rhythmic tremors of the head or trunk). Ataxia and other cerebellar symptoms may also be apparent. The diagnosis of opsoclonus-myoclonus is based on clinical, serologic, and radiographic testing. In the palliative care setting, the goals of care are always considered when deciding whether to conduct this testing.

Treatment of non-OIM myoclonus includes eliminating causative conditions. Few medications have been found to ease myoclonus. Anticonvulsants can be helpful in chronic myoclonus, although typically multidrug therapy is needed. Clonazepam is the most frequently used and most effective agent. Other drugs have been tried, including valproic acid, levetiracetam, zonisamide, acetazolamide, and sodium oxybate, although strong data for each of these medications are lacking. Several non-AEDs have been tried for myoclonus, including baclofen and dantrolene, also with varying success.

Nursing-specific care for myoclonus is multifaceted. Safety and comfort take priority:

- Padded side rails and helmets may be necessary for safety.
- For patients with severe myoclonus, ambulation may not be possible.
- Physical or occupational therapy assessment will identify whether durable medical equipment, assistive devices, or a gait belts are needed.
- Assess for pain.
- Teach patients and family members energy conservation.
- Nutritional supplementation or counseling may prevent weight loss.
- Provide a low level of stimulation (low light, minimizing noise).

Spasticity

Spasticity is increased muscle tone to the extreme. It results from denervation of muscles or from demyelination of neurons in the CNS—typically because of a lesion of the upper motor neuron. Spasticity occurs in many neurologic conditions:

- Spinal cord injury
- Multiple sclerosis (MS)
- Cerebral palsy
- Stroke

- Brain or head trauma
- Amyotrophic lateral sclerosis (ALS)
- Hereditary spastic paraplegias
- Metabolic diseases

The most sensitive indicator of an upper motor neuron lesion is a positive Babinski's sign. It is elicited by firmly stroking the lateral plantar surface of the foot. A positive Babinski's' sign is extension of the large toe accompanied by fanning and extension of the other toes during and immediately after the stimulus. Babinski's sign mimics the physiologic reflex observed in infancy. Spasticity shows a predilection for antigravity muscles: brachialis, brachioradialis, biceps, pectoralis, anterior deltoid, and the flexor carpi muscles of the arms as well as the hip flexors, gastrocnemius, hamstrings, and popliteus muscles of the legs. Other physical examination signs include hyperreflexia of the deep tendon reflexes, clonus, muscle spasms, and scissoring of extremities. Spasticity can occur in any muscle or muscle group.

Spasticity can be uncomfortable and painful. It can also severely limit functional abilities and thus requires considered treatment. The palliative care nurse will consider whether the condition is established spasticity with worsening; common causes include infection, constipation, pain, or autonomic dysreflexia. If the spasticity is new, further investigation is required. In patients with MS, the primary concern is for disease progression. It is imperative to balance spasticity with the functional abilities of the patient. For example, the patient with spastic cerebral palsy must preserve some muscle tone in order to ambulate.

Many treatments are available for spasticity. Baclofen, a γ-aminobutyric acid derivative, is the mainstay treatment. Other commonly used oral antispasmodics include dantrolene, diazepam, and tizanidine for a desired effect of diminished force of contraction. Spasticity is one of the few generally agreed on medical uses for marijuana.[5] See Table 9.5 for a summary of oral antispasmodic medications.

Phenol and botulinum toxin are injected for patients with persistent spasticity and torticollis. Surgical interventions are also available for the patient with medically intractable spasticity. Intrathecal administration of baclofen has become a mainstay of treatment for patients with persistent spasticity with significant side effects from oral baclofen. These interventions must be carefully weighed, particularly for the palliative care patient who may have limited life expectancy.

Nursing care for spasticity focuses on comfort and maximizing function. Physical and occupational therapy consultation are invaluable for prescribed stretching regimens and to determine appropriate durable medical equipment. Patient and family education are important to set realistic goals. Education also focuses on factors that worsen spasticity, prevention of pressure ulcers and contractures, fatigue, and psychosocial concerns. Early education is crucial to prevent complications. Appropriate medication use and indications for their use are also taught. Repositioning, application of heat, and strategies to improve functional abilities are helpful.

Table 9.5 Medications Used to Treat Spasticity

Drug Name	Mechanism of Action	Most Common Use	Common Side Effects
Baclofen	Inhibition of synaptic reflexes at the spinal cord level	Spasticity Hiccups	Central nervous system (CNS) depression, weakness, hypotension, gastrointestinal (GI) disturbance, polyuria
Carisoprodol	Unknown	Spasticity Muscle pain due to injury Adjunctive to opioids—use carefully in combination with any CNS depressant, especially synthetic opioids—limited use	CNS depression, idiosyncratic reactions of weakness and euphoria, seizures
Chlorzoxazone	Reduces polysynaptic reflexes	Muscle spasm and pain	Withdrawal if abruptly discontinued, CNS depression, paradoxical stimulation, GI disturbance, rash, hepatotoxicity, hypersensitivity reaction
Cyclobenzaprine	Unknown	Spasticity	CNS depression, dry mouth, dizziness, agitation
Dantrolene	Local action on the excitation-contraction units of the muscle	Spasticity Malignant hyperthermia Serotonin syndrome "Ecstasy" intoxication	CNS depression, hallucinations, hepatotoxic effects, GI disturbance
Diazepam	Reduced neuronal excitability through enhanced GABA-ergic inhibition	Agitation Alcohol detoxification Anticonvulsant Anxiolysis Spasticity Sedation	CNS depression, anterograde amnesia, psychiatric disturbance, seizures if acutely withdrawn, abuse
Gabapentin	Reduced neuronal excitability via enhanced γ-aminobutyric acid (GABA)-ergic inhibition	Anticonvulsant Neuropathic pain Spasticity	CNS depression, dizziness, weight gain, fatigue, peripheral edema, risk for suicidality

(continued)

Table 9.5 (Continued)

Orphenadrine	Anticholinergic	Low back pain, sciatica Adjuvant treatment of neuropathic pain and spasticity	CNS depression, dry mouth, dizziness, restlessness, insomnia, constipation, urine retention, orthostasis, euphoria
Metaxalone	Unknown	Muscle pain due to spasticity	CNS depression, rash, GI disturbance, leukopenia, hemolytic anemia, hepatotoxicity
Methocarbamol	Unknown	Spasticity Tetanus	CNS depression, seizures, bradycardia, syncope, hypotension, rash, GI disturbance, leukopenia, vision changes, hypersensitivity reactions
Tizanidine	Reduced neuronal excitability by α_2-adrenergic agonist	Spasticity Chronic headache Migraine	CNS depression, hepatotoxicity, sweating, GI disturbance, dry mouth, constipation, urine retention

Headaches

Headaches and migraines can be debilitating. Common conditions encountered in the palliative setting include intracranial tumors, vascular disorders, infection, and head trauma. A selection of etiologies is found in Table 9.6.

Of certain importance to the palliative care nurse is the medication overuse headache (MOH, also known as rebound headache), in which attempt at withdrawal from certain substances leads to onset of headache.[6] The typical scenario encountered in MOH is a patient using acetaminophen, nonsteroidal anti-inflammatory drugs, or a combination migraine preparation. Other identified substances include caffeine, triptans, antidepressants, cocaine, estrogen, marijuana, and opioids. The headache typically resolves in the absence of the offending substance after a period of days to weeks. In some cases, gradual reduction of dose may be a safer option, particularly if the substance has the potential for an acute withdrawal syndrome, as with opioids.

As with all neurologic changes in the palliative setting, the nurse begins with an assessment. The pain and its accompanying characteristics (intensity,

Table 9.6 Causes of Head Pain	
Headache syndromes	Cluster headache
	Tension-type headache
	Withdrawal/medication overuse headache
Migraine syndromes	Migraine with or without aura
Cranial and intracranial lesions	Metastatic brain tumors
	Primary brain tumors
	Skull base tumors
	Leptomeningeal metastases
General medical diseases and conditions	Fasting state/hunger
	Eyestrain
	Stress
	Muscle strain/tension, prolonged sitting, poor posture
	Sleep deprivation
	Stroke
	Vascular disorders
	Multiple sclerosis
	Increased intracranial pressure
	Sinus infection
	Temporal arteritis
	Varied infections, both systemic and central nervous system
Head trauma	
Atypical pain syndromes	Trigeminal neuralgia
	Post-herpetic neuralgia

location, quality, exacerbating and alleviating factors, response to previous therapies, related symptoms) can guide care.

- The typical tension-type headache is bilateral and characterized by a sensation of constant pressure.
- Episodic-type headache is thought to transform into tension-type headache with constant pericranial muscle tension. The pain can range from mild to moderate and in extreme cases can be severe.
- Migraines are commonly unilateral. The pain can be pulsatile in nature and is often associated with phonophobia, photophobia, and nausea and vomiting. Sleep alleviates the migraine, and physical activity aggravates it. A significant number of migraineurs will experience an aura of transient sensory (usually visual), language, or motor disturbance.
- Focal deficits indicate either a complex migraine or, more seriously, a new intracranial lesion.
- The "thunderclap" headache of subarachnoid hemorrhage is a sudden-onset and very severe headache often accompanied by profuse vomiting and mental status changes.
- A headache accompanied by nuchal rigidity, vomiting, and photophobia suggests irritation of the meninges and warrants emergent evaluation.

- The typical headache of a patient with intracranial metastasis is dull, poorly localized, and of moderate intensity. Some patients will have ipsilateral pain to the metastatic lesion. Signs of increased intracranial pressure include an increase in pain intensity when lying down, coughing, or sneezing as well as nausea, vomiting, mental status changes, and pupillary changes.

Physical assessment includes palpation over the area of pain. Careful neurologic examination may elicit deficits—skull base metastases will commonly compress an isolated cranial nerve. Leptomeningeal metastases will commonly result in multiple cranial or spinal neuropathies as well as headache. In some situations of headache, radiographic evaluation will be appropriate. Cerebrospinal fluid sampling by lumbar puncture may also be warranted.

Treatment is dictated by the classification of headache or migraine as well as by the etiology. Dexamethasone is commonly used in the palliative care setting of malignancy because of its oral and parental formulations, lower mineralocorticoid effects, and ease of dosing.

Nursing interventions also include patient and family education. Patients and family members benefit from education regarding pain management measures and medications. In the event of neurologic deficits, education about safety measures is important. Other nonpharmacologic interventions can be useful—ice and heat, reduced light and sound exposure, meditation and distraction, physical activity or rest, and positioning. Commonly, head-of-bed elevation is useful in the setting of increased intracranial pressure.

Impaired Communication

Communication is arguably at the heart of human existence. Impaired communication is distressing to both the patient and caregiver. Impairments in communication from neurologic disorders can take the form of aphasia, mutism, deafness, agraphia, alexia, or dysarthria. Additionally, several conditions can impede the patient's ability to express wishes—the ventilator-dependent patient is one such example. The patient with a massive brainstem injury from a basilar artery occlusion is "locked in" and has retained cognitive abilities but lost all control of the body save for voluntary eye movement.

Nursing care for the patient with disorders of speech or language focuses on strategizing alternative means of communication and maximizing functional ability for speech. Impaired communication is highly distressing and frustrating for patients and caregivers alike. If the patient is capable of cognition, the nurse identifies alternative communication strategies regardless of the patient's prognosis and the setting of care. Communication boards, yes/no questions, and written instructions are useful. Several key points are important for the patient with aphasia (Box 9.3).

Speech-language pathology consultation can be immensely helpful to clarify the specific communication deficiencies. Speech pathologists are a wonderful resource to the palliative care nurse for strategizing alternative communication methods. Song may be used for the patient with expressive aphasia to communicate because some patients with nonfluent aphasia may be able to put words to familiar melody in order to communicate.

Box 9.3 Key Points for Optimizing Communication

Provide the optimal setting for communication: Ensure the patient has glasses on and hearing aids in, if appropriate, and adequate lighting.

Avoid correcting grammatical mistakes or speaking for the patient.

Do not raise the volume of your voice unless the patient is hearing impaired.

Use facial expression to emphasize spoken communication.

Face the patient directly while communicating.

If the patient has other neurologic impairment, such as a visual field cut, compensate by standing on the patient's best side.

Simplify the message.

Allow adequate time for cognitive processing and response.

A technique known as melodic intonation therapy has been developed for patients with left-hemisphere lesions to increase length of spoken phrases. Music therapy has a potential role as well for the patient with communication difficulty.

Management of Specific Neurologic Degenerative Disorders

A number of neurologic diseases result in devastating symptom clusters and require increasingly complex nursing care. Many of these diseases are progressive neurologic degenerative disorders such as ALS, MS, and Parkinson's disease (PD). This section will address the palliative care needs of these patients.

Amyotrophic Lateral Sclerosis

ALS, also known as Lou Gehrig's disease, is a devastating progressive neurologic condition characterized by progressive muscle wasting from denervation (amyotrophy) with hyperreflexia. ALS is the most common of all motor neuron diseases. ALS results from the destruction of both upper and lower motor neurons. The end result of the disease process is paralysis and respiratory failure, and as a result, fear and psychological distress underlie the diagnosis. Table 9.7 highlights the typical symptom clusters of ALS.

Goals-of-care discussions are important early in the disease trajectory.[7] Median life expectancy is less than 5 years, although life expectancy is

---

Table 9.7 Symptoms Common to the Patient With Amyotrophic Lateral Sclerosis

Bulbar Onset	Limb Onset
Dysphagia	Muscle weakness
Dysarthria	Hyperreflexia
Sialorrhea	Fasciculations

considerably shorter if the patient declines artificial nutritional or respiratory support. The ALS patient requires an extensive team. Neurologists, pulmonologists, speech pathologists, physical and occupational therapists, nurses, and social workers will all play a role.

Nursing interventions for the patient with ALS are critical and focus on quality of life, symptom palliation, and functional ability as well as end-of-life planning and support (Table 9.8).

Parkinson's Disease

PD is the second most common neurologic degenerative disorder. Related conditions include multiple system atrophy and progressive supranuclear palsy. The defining characteristics of PD are tremor, postural instability, bradykinesia, and rigidity of the extremities or trunk.

A summary of available medical treatments can be found in Box 9.4. The medication regimens for PD can be complex, and doses are terrifically time sensitive because of the rapid onset and offset of activity of

Table 9.8 Nursing Management of Amyotrophic Lateral Sclerosis

Airway and secretions	
Sialorrhea (excessive saliva in the oral cavity)	Anticholinergics—use with care because of risk for mucous plugging, orthostasis, confusion, sedation
	Glycopyrrolate, amitriptyline, atropine, benztropine mesylate, trihexyphenidyl, hyoscyamine, transdermal scopolamine
	Radiation to salivary gland
	Botulinum toxin to parotid gland
Mucous pooling	Suction
	Cough-assist device
	Guaifenesin
	β-Blockers
Airway	Noninvasive ventilation, such as positive-pressure ventilation with continuous positive airway pressure, bilevel positive airway pressure
Note: Early discussion of goals of care and patient preferences is required.	Tracheostomy with or without long-term mechanical ventilation
	Oxygen support
	Positioning
Communication impairment	Speech-language pathologist evaluation
	Alphabet boards, picture board, yes/no board
	Electronic equipment if appropriate
Pseudobulbar affect (PBA)	Selective serotonin reuptake inhibitors
Note: PBA is not a mood disorder, but a separate mood disorder may underlie the PBA.	Tricyclic antidepressants
	Dextromethorphan/quinidine

(continued)

Table 9.8 (Continued)

Falls, loss of mobility	Early physical and occupational therapy referral
	Home nursing referral
	Durable medical equipment
	Assistive devices
	Stretching, range-of-motion exercises
	Positioning exercises
	Anticipating toileting needs
	Energy-sparing strategies
Spasticity, cramps, amyotrophic lateral sclerosis (ALS)-specific pain *Note:* Pain is common in ALS.	Opioids
	Nonopioids
	Balancing opioids with concerns for tenuous respiratory status and patient preferences
Mood disorder, anxiety *Note:* Strategies for managing requests for euthanasia and assisted suicide are required.	Evaluate increased risk for suicide, suicidal ideation
	Treat underlying depression, anxiety
Nutrition	Changes in food and liquid consistency
	Smaller, more frequent meals
	Ensuring solid foods are soft and moist
	Using straws, chin-tuck maneuver if appropriate
	Gastrostomy tube if consistent with patient's preferences
Cognitive changes	Frontotemporal dementia, although an unusual presentation, can occur in ALS patients
	Managing dementia behaviors
Terminal phase of ALS *Note:* Early discussion with patients and caregivers about when to refer to hospice is required.	Highly aggressive symptom management
	Palliative sedation has been explored for patients with ALS

most levodopa-containing medications. One key point is the potential for diminished drug absorption when PD medications are taken with protein-rich meals.

The palliative care nurse will be initially focused on maximizing functional ability and diminishing falls (Table 9.9). Medication education, home safety, physical and occupational therapy, and establishing a routine of exercise and rest are important goals of nursing care.[8] Because PD and the dopaminomimetic therapies can result in a degree of autonomic instability, the nurse will evaluate for hypotensive episodes and gastrointestinal dysmotility. The speech therapist also has a role in the evaluation of the patient with PD—dysphagia, impaired communication, drooling, and aspiration are common. Fluctuating energy expenditure, medication-food interactions, impaired gastrointestinal motility, and fluid imbalance leave patients with PD at risk for nutritional deficiencies.[9] As a result, the nutritionist has a role across the disease trajectory for the patient with PD. The psychosocial needs of the patient with PD and the family must be addressed. The nurse assesses

Box 9.4 Medications Commonly Used for Movement Disorders in Parkinson's Disease

Levodopa and Levodopa-Modifying Drugs

Mechanism of action

Dosing schedule

Rationale: increase survival and quality of life

Adverse effects: nausea and vomiting, psychosis, compulsive behaviors

Reduced bioavailability of levodopa/carbidopa (LC) and levodopa/benserazide (LB) when taken with protein-rich meals

Catechol-O-Methyl Transferase Inhibitors

Mechanism of action: decrease metabolism of levodopa

Increase the half-life of levodopa, LC, LB, simultaneously increasing efficacy of doses

Available as entacapone and tolcapone

Lead to longer "on" periods and shorter "off" periods

Notably do not decrease the dyskinesia effects of levodopa

Monoamine Oxidase Inhibitors

Dopamine metabolizer

Can reduce the needed dose of levodopa by 30% to 40%

Dopamine Antagonists

Often used for initial treatment

Lower risk for causing dyskinesia

Available in extended-release formulations

Shortened "off" time compared with levodopa

Risk for compulsive behaviors such as gambling, hypersexual behavior, and eating disorders

Available in oral formulations, as continuous subcutaneous infusion, or as continuous duodenal infusion through portable mini-pump

Apomorphine injection for sudden "off" periods

Table 9.9 Nursing Care in Parkinson's Disease

Fatigue, falls, loss of independence	Referral for physical, occupational, or dance therapy
	Tai-chi to improve balance
	Home modifications
	Home nursing evaluation
	Durable medical equipment evaluation
	Evaluation for hypotensive episodes
Communication and swallowing disorders	Impaired facial expression ("masked face") further impairs functioning
	Assess for pseudobulbar affect if expressed mood and affect are discongruent

for depression, anxiety, and caregiver distress. Grief, feelings of loss, and uncertainty of the future are common. Financial concerns and social isolation should also be addressed.

The terminal phase of PD is typically heralded by progressive loss of mobility, worsening dysphagia, and aspiration. PD-associated dementia can occur as well. The palliative care nurse will expand the goals of nursing intervention to include continence care, preserving patient preferences, managing medication effects, and patient and family education about symptoms at the end of life.

Huntington's Disease

Huntington's disease (HD) is characterized by a classic triad—dementia, choreoathetosis, and autosomal dominant inheritance. It is a devastating disease with all-encompassing effects on the patient and family. Indeed, the family is often familiar with the disease—typically, a family will have affected members across several generations. Patients are usually diagnosed in the third through the fifth decades of life, although juvenile-onset HD is well established. Identification of the causative gene has allowed recent generations to make informed life decisions. There is also a psychological burden of knowing that one will die of a devastating neurologic disease. The ideal setting for the HD patient is in a multidisciplinary clinic that includes nurses with palliative care training. Affected patients ultimately require care with all personal needs.

Palliative care nursing for the patient with HD ideally begins with early identification. There is currently no cure for HD. Symptoms must be treated carefully. The most outwardly obvious symptom is the movement disorder. Notably, the chorea may not be bothersome to the patient and should be treated only if it is functionally impairing to the patient. Treating the chorea must be done carefully and ideally with the assistance of a skilled neurologist. Dopamine-blocking agents and dopamine-depleting agents are both used.

Psychiatric disorders in HD are common and highly disabling. The cognitive dysfunction is progressive, but the psychiatric symptoms are typically static. Cognitive dysfunction typically precedes the onset of motor symptoms and evolves into full dementia. The neurocognitive effects of HD are characterized by bradyphrenia, poor spatial memory, diminished working memory, impaired capacity for planning, poor judgment, and decreased mental flexibility. Psychiatric disturbances range from emotional lability and behavior disorder to major mood disorder, suicidality, and homicidality.

As HD progresses, chorea progresses until the patient is unable to be still for more than a few moments at a time. Eventually, chorea gives way to a hypokinetic, abulic state and then to a vegetative state. Muscles become rigid. Patients may experience tremor, bradykinesia, and dysphagia. Many patients will be placed in residential facilities by this stage. Nursing care involves safety assessment, positioning, and feeding assistance. Patients commonly suffer pain from falls, injuries, and hyperkinetic movements. Table 9.10 lists important nursing interventions for these patients.

Table 9.10 Symptomatic Treatment of Huntington's Disease	
Chorea	Treat carefully and only if distressing to the patient or functionally impairing
	Haloperidol 2–10 mg/day
	Olanzapine has been found to reduce chorea, stabilize mood, and augment antidepressants; may also improve ambulation
	Tetrabenazine improves motor function and suppresses chorea; monitor closely for parkinsonism, mood disorder, suicidality, sedation, akathisia
Parkinson's disease	Treated with standard Parkinson's therapy
	Poor candidates for neurosurgical interventions
	Often characterized by rigidity in the terminal stages of disease
Bruxism	Separate from the effects of neuroleptics
	Well-managed with botulinum toxin
Dystonia	May be painful
	Functionally impairing
	No specific treatment has been evaluated in trials
Aggressive behavior, mood disorder	Antidepressants
	Antipsychotics
	Propranolol
	Mood stabilizers
	Buspirone
	Suicidal and homicidal assessment
Sleep-wake cycle disruption	Significant circadian rhythm disturbance
	Insomnia is not the dominant feature
	Although efficacy is not established, scheduled hypnotics are reported in the literature

Certainly, the most difficult task is supporting the patient and family through the inevitable decline. Emotional support and evaluation for mood disorder will be ongoing tasks for the nurse. Family and caregiver education will focus on the disease process and the risk for potentially affected family members. Early discussions about end-of-life preferences are also important.

Multiple Sclerosis

MS is a neuroimmunologic disease with widely varying symptoms, is typically diagnosed in young to middle adulthood, and is more commonly found in people of northern European decent and those living farther from the Equator. Although no cure exists for MS at the present, much can be done to alleviate the symptom burden. Cognitive dysfunction is seen in severe disease. Patients describe disabling fatigue, functional impairments, bowel and bladder dysfunction, and sexual dysfunction, among others. Managing disability is at the heart of nursing interventions for the patient with MS (Table 9.11). Mobility and independent activities of daily living typically decline as the disease progresses. Early and scheduled physical and occupational therapy assessments are wise. Home and workplace modifications can preserve the

Table 9.11 Managing Symptoms of Multiple Sclerosis

Fatigue	Neurostimulants
	Amantadine
	Regular exercise
	Planned rest breaks, energy-sparing techniques
Cognitive dysfunction	Neuropsychological assessment
Neurogenic bladder: urinary frequency, urgency, bladder spasticity, incomplete emptying	Urinary retention: bethanechol, intermittent catheterization; monitor and treat high postvoid residual volumes to reduce risk for urinary tract infection
	Frequency and urgency: propantheline, oxybutynin
Sexual dysfunction	Men: phosphodiesterase type 5 inhibitors
Pain	Pain assessment
	Traditional methods of pain control can be effective, especially neuroleptics, gabapentin, and tricyclic antidepressants
Tremor	Severe postural tremor can respond to isoniazid with pyridoxine
	Carbamazepine
	Clonazepam
	Light weights applied to the wrists
Neurogenic bowel	Prescribed bowel program of:
	Scheduled toileting (especially after eating or exercising)
	Stool softeners, laxatives, suppositories, enemas if needed
	Digital rectal stimulation if needed
Mood disorder	Aggressive management of depression
	Referral for neuropsychological testing

patient's functional independence. As with most incurable diseases, emotional support is frequently necessary.

Myasthenia Gravis

Myasthenia gravis (MG) is a life-threatening neuroimmunologic disease. The disease stems from the destruction of acetylcholine receptors at the neuromuscular junction. The common presentation is a patient with fluctuating weakness of the muscles, especially the muscles innervated by brainstem motor neurons. Weakness can be induced with repetitive movement, and strength is restored with rest. Strength is characteristically restored dramatically with anticholinesterase drugs. MG was once a fatal disease shortly after diagnosis. Although there is no cure for MG, the discovery of anticholinesterase-inhibiting medications has allowed many patients with MG to pursue full lives.

Symptom control focuses on managing and preventing acute MG crisis. During crisis, palliative management focuses on symptoms of dyspnea and anxiety. In the long-term care of patients with MG, careful discussions about intubation and the possibility of prolonged mechanical ventilation are warranted. Some patients will ultimately require tracheostomy.

Table 9.12 Symptoms of Intracranial Lesion by Location

Structure	Normal Function	Altered Function in the Presence of Tumor
Frontal lobe	Personality	Personality change or disinhibition
	Voluntary skeletal movements	Altered responses to stimuli, emotional lability
	Fine repetitive motor movements	Difficulty with speaking, chewing, or facial expressions
	Eye movements	Uncoordinated swallowing, or movement of hands, arms, torso, pelvis, legs, and feet
Parietal lobe	Sensory processing: tactile, visual, gustatory, olfactory, auditory, body position	Trouble integrating language, vision, and tactile stimuli
		Loss of sense of body positioning or vibratory sense
		Difficulty with verbal and nonverbal memory
		Paresthesias
		Loss of tactile discrimination
		Inability to write or do math calculations
Occipital lobe	Interpretation of visual input	Difficulty naming visual images and words
		Difficulty reading and writing, identifying colors
		Inability to identify if an object is moving
Temporal lobe	Auditory perception and interpretation	*Right lobe:*
		Difficulty hearing, understanding, organizing, and concentrating on what is seen or heard
		Inability to recognize musical tones and nonspeech information like illustrations
		Olfactory or gustatory hallucinations
		Vertigo, unsteadiness, or tinnitus
		Left lobe:
		Difficulty hearing, understanding, organizing, and concentrating on what is seen or heard
		Inability to recognize spoken words
		Vertigo, unsteadiness, or tinnitus

(continued)

Table 9.12 (Continued)

Cerebellum	Processing of sensory information from eyes, ears, tactile and musculoskeletal receptors Refining motor activity into coordinated movement	Frequent loss of balance, unstable posture or gait Uncoordinated movement of extremities Alterations of some reflexive movements Nystagmus, muscle tremors, or ataxia
Brainstem and cranial nerves (CNs)	*Brainstem:* gateway from cerebrum and cerebellum to spinal cord. Maintains consciousness, cardiovascular and respiratory functioning Relays motor and sensory information *Cranial nerves:* Nuclei of CN III to CN XII arise within the brainstem structures	CN I: loss of smell (anosmia) CN II: vision compromise, visual field defect CN III: loss of pupillary constriction and ability to raise eyelid, loss of extraocular movements, diplopia CN IV: loss of inferior/medial eye movement CN V: inability to clench jaw and chew, numbness of mouth and nose, numbness of face, loss of corneal reflex CN VI: inability to abduct the eye CN VII: facial paralysis, taste disturbance, salivary and lacrimal dysfunction CN VIII: loss of hearing, disequilibrium CN IX: swallowing difficulty, taste disturbance CN X: loss of ear sensation, gastrointestinal disturbance, voice hoarseness CN XI: difficulty turning head and shrugging shoulders CN XII: difficulty swallowing and articulating lingual sounds

Intracranial Lesions

Intracranial tumors encompass both primary and metastatic tumors and may involve cerebrospinal fluid, bony structures of the skull and skull base, dura, and cranial nerves. Cancers that commonly metastasize to the CNS are lung, melanoma, renal cell, breast, and colorectal. The most common primary CNS tumors include meningioma, the gliomas, embryonal tumors such as medulloblastoma, and primary CNS lymphoma. The palliative care goals will be different for patients with widely metastatic cancer, newly diagnosed intracranial metastases but stable system disease, or primary CNS tumors. A thoughtful discussion with the oncologist can be immensely helpful for the nurse in any of these settings. Symptoms of intracranial lesions vary widely by location of tumor (Table 9.12).

Treatment for the palliative care patient typically incorporates high-potency corticosteroids. Corticosteroids restore the blood-brain barrier by reducing the permeability of vascular endothelial cells and thus reducing intracranial pressure. Steroids can alleviate headache and pain from metastases. Seizure management, discussed previously, may be warranted, although prophylactic AEDs have not been found useful to prevent their onset. Nursing care begins with assessment of comfort, safety, communication, and many other variables; interventions are then incorporated based on patient and family needs.

Conclusion

Arguably, the role of the palliative care nurse is first to alleviate suffering and second to advocate for the patient's choices. The task of assisting the patient to identify his or her health care choices in the face of a devastating and often terminal neurologic illness is not an easy one. Several other themes emerge, including advocating for early therapy referral, pain control, bowel and bladder care, preserving functional abilities, maintaining patients' independence, and providing education about medications and disease processes.

References

1. Hauser WA, Beghi E. First seizure definitions and worldwide incidence and mortality. *Epilepsia*. 2008;49(Suppl 1):8–12.

2. Gretton SK, Ross JR, Rutter D, et al. Plasma morphine and metabolite concentrations are associated with clinical effects of morphine in cancer patients. *J Pain Symptom Manage*. 2013;45(4):670–680.

3. Cherny N, Ripamonti C, Pereira J, et al; Expert Working Group of the European Association of Palliative Care Network. Strategies to manage the adverse effects of oral morphine: an evidence-based report. *J Clin Oncol*. 2001;19(9):2542–2554.

4. Stone P, Minton O. European Palliative Care Research collaborative pain guidelines. Central side-effects management: what is the evidence to support best practice in the management of sedation, cognitive impairment and myoclonus? *Palliat Med*. 2011;25(5):431–441.

5. Corey-Bloom J, Wolfson T, Gamst A, et al. Smoked cannabis for spasticity in multiple sclerosis: a randomized placebo-controlled trial. *CMAJ*. 2012;184(10):1 143–1150.

6. Rapaport AM. Medication overuse headache: awareness, detection and treatment. *CNS Drugs*. 2008;22(12):995–1004.

7. Mitsumoto H, Rabkin JG. Palliative care for patients with amyotrophic lateral sclerosis: "Prepare for the worst and hope for the best." *JAMA*. 2007;298(2):207–215.

8. Li F, Harmer P, Fitzgerald K, et al. Tai chi and postural stability in patients with Parkinson's disease. *N Engl J Med*. 2012;366(6):511–519.

9. Barichella M, Cereda E, Pezzoli G. Major nutritional issues in the management of Parkinson's disease. *Mov Disord*. 2009;24(13):1881–1892.

Chapter 10

Anxiety and Depression

Jeannie V. Pasacreta, Pamela A. Minarik, Leslie Nield-Anderson, and Judith A. Paice

Introduction

This chapter provides information regarding the assessment and treatment of anxiety and depression among individuals faced with chronic or life-threatening illness, and delineates psychosocial interventions that are effective at minimizing these troubling symptoms. Practical guidelines regarding patient management and identifying patients who may require formal psychiatric consultation are offered.

Changes in Health Care That Have Accentuated Psychiatric Symptoms

Changes in health care delivery and rapid scientific gains are simultaneously increasing the number of individuals receiving or in need of palliative care at any given time, the longevity and course of chronic diseases, and the prevalence and intensity of the psychological symptoms that accompany them.[1,2] Furthermore, psychological distress is experienced within an increasingly complex, fragmented, and impersonal health care system that tends to intensify these symptoms. Despite these realities, psychological symptoms receive minimal attention, and health care providers often lack the needed education and support regarding assessment, treatment, and referral of these common problems.

Individuals are being diagnosed earlier and living longer, with increasing opportunities to experience simultaneous, interrelated psychosocial and medical comorbidity. Concurrent treatment discoveries have increased quantity of life, albeit with ill-defined consequences to quality of life.[2]

Soaring medical costs, managed care arrangements, and the stigma associated with mental illness have simultaneously placed a low priority on the recognition and treatment of psychosocial distress within our health care system.

Lack of assessment and treatment of the common psychiatric sequelae to chronic disease have been linked to such problems as treatment-resistant depression and anxiety, family dysfunction, lack of compliance with prevention and treatment recommendations, potentiation of physical symptoms, and suicide.

In dealing with depressed and/or anxious patients referred for evaluation, the decision to intervene with psychotherapy or pharmacologic agents may be based largely on the philosophy, educational background, and past experience of individual clinicians.

Patients who exhibit depressive or anxious symptoms not considered severe enough to classify for "psychiatric" status are frequently not offered psychotherapeutic services, and the natural history of their symptoms is rarely monitored over time.

Because depression and anxiety are common among individuals with chronic illness, recognition and management of these symptoms is extremely important, particularly because they are often responsive to treatment. Patients, family, and professional caregivers need to be informed of the factors that affect psychological adjustment, the wide range of psychological responses that accompany chronic and progressive disease, and the efficacy of various modes of intervention.

The Clinical Course of Chronic Illness

Acute stress is a common response to the diagnosis of a life-threatening illness and resurfaces at transitional points in the disease process (beginning treatment, recurrence, treatment failure, disease progression).[3] The response is characterized by shock, disbelief, anxiety, depression, sleep and appetite disturbance, and difficulty performing activities of daily living. Under favorable circumstances, these psychological symptoms should resolve within a short period. The time period is variable, but consensus is that after the crisis has passed and the individual knows what to expect in terms of a treatment plan, psychological symptoms diminish. Patients who are diagnosed with late-stage disease or who have aggressive illnesses with no hope for cure are often most vulnerable to psychological distress—particularly anxiety, depression, family problems, and physical discomfort.

Diagnostic Phase

The period from time of diagnosis through initiation of a treatment plan is characterized by medical evaluation, the development of new relationships with unfamiliar medical personnel, and the need to integrate a barrage of information that, at best, is frightening and confusing. Patients and families frequently experience a heightened sense of responsibility, worry, and isolation during this period. They are particularly anxious and fearful when receiving initial information regarding diagnosis and treatment. Consequently, care should be taken by professionals to repeat information over several sessions and to inquire about patients' and families' understanding of the facts and treatment options.

During the diagnostic period, patient concerns commonly focus on existential issues of life and death, rather than on concerns related to health, work, finances, religion, self, or relationships with family and friends. Early assessment by clinicians can help to identify individuals at risk for later adjustment problems or psychiatric disorders and in the greatest need of ongoing psychosocial support.[3]

The initial response to diagnosis may be profoundly influenced by a person's prior association with a particular disease. Those with memories of close relatives with the same illness often demonstrate heightened distress, particularly if the relative died or had negative treatment experiences. During the diagnostic period, patients may search for explanations or causes for their disease and may struggle to give personal meaning to their experience. Ongoing involvement and accurate information will minimize uncertainty and the development of maladaptive coping strategies based on erroneous beliefs.

Although the literature substantiates the devastating emotional impact of a life-threatening chronic illness, it also well documents that many individuals cope effectively. Positive coping strategies, such as taking action and finding favorable characteristics in the situation, have been reported to be effective. Contrary to the beliefs of many clinicians, denial also has been found to assist patients in coping effectively, unless sustained and used excessively to a point that it interferes with appropriate treatment.

Recurrence and Progressive Disease

Development of a recurrence after a disease-free interval can be especially devastating for patients and those close to them. Shock and depression are not uncommon after relapse and require individuals and their families to reevaluate the future. This period is a difficult one, during which patients may also experience pessimism, renewed preoccupation with death and dying, and feelings of helplessness and disenchantment with the medical system. As a disease progresses, the person frequently reports an upsetting scenario that includes frequent pain, disability, increased dependence on others, and diminished functional ability, which then potentiates psychological symptoms. As uncomfortable symptoms increase, perceived quality of life diminishes. Thus, an important goal in the psychosocial treatment of patients with advanced chronic illness focuses on symptom control.

An issue that repeatedly surfaces among patients, family members, and professional care providers deals with the use of aggressive treatment protocols in the presence of progressive disease. Often, patients and families request to participate in experimental protocols even when there is little likelihood of extending survival. Controversy continues about the efficacy of such therapies and the role health professionals can play in facilitating patients' choices about participating. These issues become even more important because changes in the health care system may limit payment for costly and highly technical treatments.

It is essential for health care professionals to establish structured dialogue with patients, family members, and care providers regarding treatment goals and expectations. Despite the existence of progressive illness, certain individuals may respond to investigational treatment with increased hope.

Efforts to separate and clarify values, thoughts, and emotional reactions of care providers, patients, and families to these delicate issues are important if individualized care with attention to psychological symptoms is to be provided.

Use of resources such as psychiatric consultation-liaison nurses, psychiatrists, psychologists, social workers, and chaplains can be invaluable in assisting patients, family members, and staff to grapple with these issues in a meaningful and productive manner.

Terminal Disease and Dying

When the terminal period has begun, it is usually not the fact of dying but the quality of dying that is the overwhelming issue confronting the patient and family.[4] Continued palliative care into the terminal stage of cancer relieves physical and psychological symptoms, promotes comfort, and increases well-being.

Patients living in the final phase of any advanced chronic illness experience fears and anxiety related to uncertain future events, such as unrelieved pain, separation from loved ones, burden on family, and loss of control. Psychological distress is more likely in persons confronting diminished life span, physical debilitation associated with functional limitation, or symptoms associated with toxic therapies. Therapeutic interventions should be directed toward increasing patients' sense of control and self-efficacy within the context of functional decline and increased dependence.

Personal values and beliefs, socioeconomic and cultural background, and religious belief systems influence patients' expectations about quality of life and palliative care. Awareness of the family system's cultural, religious, ethnic, and socioeconomic background is important to the understanding of their beliefs, attitudes, practices, and behaviors related to illness and death.

Delirium, depression, suicidal ideation, and severe anxiety are among the most common psychiatric complications encountered in terminally ill cancer patients.[5] Psychiatric emergencies require the same rapid intervention as distressing physical symptoms and medical crises. Despite the seemingly overwhelming nature of psychosocial responses along the chronic illness trajectory, most patients do indeed cope effectively. Periods of intense emotions, such as anxiety and depression, are not necessarily the same as maladaptive coping.

Factors That Affect Psychological Adjustment

Psychological responses to chronic illness vary widely and are influenced by many individual factors. Three of the most important factors are previous coping strategies and emotional stability, social support, and symptom distress. In addition, there are common medical conditions, treatments, and substances that may cause or intensify symptoms of anxiety and depression (Tables 10.1 and 10.2).

Previous Coping Strategies and Emotional Stability

One of the most important predictors of psychological adjustment to chronic illness is the emotional stability and coping strategies used by the person before diagnosis. Individuals with a history of poor psychological adjustment

Table 10.1 Common Medical Conditions Associated With Anxiety and Depression

Anxiety	Depression
• Endocrine disorders: hyperthyroidism and hypothyroidism, hyperglycemia and hypoglycemia, Cushing's disease, carcinoid syndrome, pheochromocytoma	• Cardiovascular: cardiovascular disease, congestive heart failure, myocardial infarct, cardiac arrhythmias
	• Central nervous system: cerebrovascular accident, cerebral anoxia, Huntington's disease, subdural hematoma, Alzheimer's disease, HIV infection, dementia, carotid stenosis, temporal lobe epilepsy, multiple sclerosis, postconcussion syndrome, myasthenia gravis, narcolepsy, subarachnoid hemorrhage
• Cardiovascular conditions: myocardial infarction, paroxysmal atrial tachycardia, angina pectoris, congestive heart failure, mitral valve prolapse, hypovolemia	
• Metabolic conditions: hyperkalemia, hypercalcemia, hypoglycemia, hyperthermia, anemia, hyponatremia	
• Respiratory conditions: asthma, chronic obstructive pulmonary disease, pneumonia, pulmonary edema, pulmonary embolus, respiratory dependence, hypoxia	• Autoimmune: rheumatoid arthritis, polyarteritis nodosa
	• Endocrine: hyperparathyroidism, hypothyroidism, diabetes mellitus, Cushing's disease, Addison's disease
• Neoplasms: islet cell adenomas, pheochromocytoma	• Other: alcoholism, anemia, systemic lupus erythematosus, Epstein-Barr virus, hepatitis, malignancies, pulmonary insufficiency, pancreatic or liver disease, syphilis, encephalitis, malnutrition
• Neurologic conditions: akathisia, encephalopathy, seizure disorder, vertigo, mass lesion, postconcussion syndrome	

Adapted from references 3 to 5.

Table 10.2 Common Medications and Substances Associated With Anxiety and Depression

Anxiety	Depression
Alcohol and nicotine withdrawal	Antihypertensives
Stimulants, including caffeine	Analgesics
Thyroid replacement	Antiparkinsonian agents
Neuroleptics	Hypoglycemic agents
Corticosteroids	Steroids
Sedative-hypnotic withdrawal or paradoxical reaction	Chemotherapeutic agents
Bronchodilators and decongestants	Estrogen and progesterone
Cocaine	Antimicrobials
Epinephrine	L-dopa
Benzodiazepines and their withdrawal	Benzodiazepines
Digitalis toxicity	Barbiturates
Cannabis	Alcohol
Antihypertensives	Phenothiazines
Antihistamines	Amphetamines
Antiparkinsonian medications	Lithium carbonate
Oral contraceptives	Heavy metals
Anticholinergics	Cimetidine
Anesthetics and analgesics	Antibiotics
Toxins	
Antidepressants	

Adapted from references 3 to 5.

and of clinically significant anxiety or depression are at highest risk for emotional decompensation and should be monitored closely throughout all phases of treatment. This is particularly true for people with a history of major psychiatric syndromes and/or psychiatric hospitalization.

Social Support

Social support consistently has been found to influence a person's psychosocial adjustment to chronic illness. The ability and availability of significant others in dealing with diagnosis and treatment can significantly affect the patient's view of himself or herself and potentially the patient's survival. Individuals who are able to maintain close connections with family and friends during the course of illness are more likely to cope effectively with the disease than those who are not able to maintain such relationships.

Symptom Distress

The effects of treatment for a variety of chronic diseases, as well as the impact of progressive illness, can inflict transient or permanent physical changes, physical symptom distress, and functional impairments in patients. Excessive psychological distress can exacerbate the side effects of cancer treatment agents, and conversely, treatment side effects can have a dramatic impact on the psychological profiles of patients.[6] As uncomfortable symptoms increase, perceived quality of life diminishes and psychiatric symptoms often worsen. The presence of increased physical discomfort, combined with a lack of control and predictability regarding the occurrence of symptoms, amplifies anxiety, depression, and organic mental symptoms in patients with advanced disease.

Differentiating Psychiatric Complications From Expected Psychological Responses

Differentiating between symptoms related to a medical illness and symptoms related to an underlying psychiatric disorder is particularly challenging to health care practitioners.

Anxiety and depression are normal responses to life events and illness and occur throughout the palliative care trajectory. Symptoms following stressful events in a person's life (employment difficulties, retirement, death of a family member, loss of a job, diagnosis of a medical or life-threatening illness) are expected to dissipate as an individual copes, with reassurance and validation from family and friends, and adapts to the situation.

When responses predominantly include excessive nervousness, worry, and fear, diagnosis of an adjustment disorder with anxiety is applied. If an individual responds with tearfulness and feelings of hopelessness, he or she is characterized as experiencing an adjustment disorder with depressed mood. An adjustment disorder with mixed anxiety and depressed mood is characterized by a combination of both anxiety and depression.

Referrals from primary care providers for psychiatric assistance with psychopharmacologic treatment are indicated when symptoms continue, intensify, or disrupt an individual's life beyond a 6-month period or when symptoms do not respond to conventional reassurance and validation by the primary care provider and support from an individual's social network.

Most patients develop transient psychological symptoms that are responsive to support, reassurance, and information about what to expect regarding a disease course and its treatment. There are some individuals, however, who require more aggressive psychotherapeutic intervention, such as pharmacotherapy and ongoing psychotherapy.

Guidelines to Help Clinicians Identify Patients Who Exhibit Behavior That Suggests the Presence of a Psychiatric Syndrome

If the patient's problems become so severe that supportive measures are insufficient to control emotional distress, referral to a psychiatric clinician is indicated. Factors that may predict major psychiatric problems along the chronic illness trajectory include past psychiatric hospitalization; history of significant depression, manic-depressive illness, schizophrenia, organic mental conditions, or personality disorders; lack of social support; inadequate control of physical discomfort; history of or current alcohol and/or drug abuse; and currently prescribed psychotropic medication.

The need for psychiatric referral among patients receiving psychotropic medication deserves specific mention because it is often overlooked in clinical practice. Standard therapies used to treat major chronic diseases, such as surgery and chemotherapy, and/or disease progression itself can significantly change dosage requirements for medications used to treat major psychiatric syndromes such as anxiety, depression, and bipolar disorder. For example, dosage requirements for lithium carbonate, commonly used to treat the manic episodes associated with bipolar disorder and the depressive episodes associated with recurrent depressive disorder, can change significantly over the course of treatment for a number of chronic diseases. Therapeutic blood levels of lithium are closely tied to sodium and water balance. Additionally, lithium has a narrow therapeutic window, and life-threatening toxicity can develop rapidly. Treatment side effects such as diarrhea, fever, vomiting, and resulting dehydration warrant scrupulous monitoring of dosage and side effects.

Careful monitoring is also indicated during preoperative and postoperative periods. Another common problem among patients treated with psychotropic medication is that medications may be discontinued at specific points in the treatment process, such as the time of surgery, and not restarted.

For some patients, psychological distress does not subside with the usual supportive interventions. Unfortunately, clinically relevant and severe psychiatric syndromes may go unrecognized by nonpsychiatric care providers. One of the reasons that it may be difficult to detect serious anxiety and depression in patients is that several of the diagnostic criteria used to evaluate their presence, such as lack of appetite, insomnia, decreased sexual interest, psychomotor agitation, and diminished energy, may overlap with usual disease and treatment effects.

The Coexisting Nature of Psychiatric and Medical Symptoms

Depression and anxiety are appropriate to the stress of having a serious illness, and the boundary between normal and abnormal symptoms is often unclear. Even when diagnostic criteria are met for a major depressive episode or anxiety disorder, there is disagreement regarding the need for psychiatric treatment because psychiatric symptoms may improve on initiation of medical treatment. A major source of diagnostic confusion is the overlap of somatic symptoms associated with several chronic illnesses and their treatments and symptoms pathognomonic to depression and anxiety themselves (e.g., fatigue, loss of appetite, weakness, weight loss, restlessness, agitation). Separating out whether a symptom is due to depression, anxiety, the medical illness and its treatment, or a combination of factors is often exceedingly difficult.

Anxiety or Depression With a Medical or Pharmacologic Etiology

During progressive or active treatment phases of a chronic disease, symptoms of anxiety or depression may recur at various intervals relative to a specific causative agent, the stress associated with the illness, or a combination of those and other factors. Physical and medication history, mental status, psychosocial and psychiatric histories (see Box 10.1 for screening instruments), electrocardiogram, comprehensive laboratory tests including toxicology screening, relevant family information regarding available support systems, and changes in lifestyle and functioning all will promote accurate assessment and close monitoring throughout the palliative care trajectory.[7]

Individuals experiencing depression do not always present with a dysphoric effect or report distressing feelings of hopelessness and helplessness. Instead, they may present with somatic complaints such as dizziness, headaches, excessive fatigue, sleep disturbances, or irritability. Disturbances in appetite, sleep, energy, and concentration are hallmark symptoms of depression. However, in medically ill people, these symptoms are frequently caused by the medical illness. Symptoms such as fearfulness, depressed appearance, social withdrawal, brooding, self-pity, pessimism, a sense of punishment, and mood that cannot be changed (e.g., cannot be cheered up, not smiling, does not respond to good news) are considered to be more reliable.

Boxes 10.2 and 10.3 list general criteria to diagnose an anxiety and depressive disorder in medically ill people.[3,5] Whenever symptoms are unremitting or intensify and do not respond to conventional professional and family support, psychiatric evaluations for psychopharmacologic and psychotherapeutic interventions are warranted.

Anxiety or Depression Precipitated by a Medical Disorder

In many cases, an anxiety or depressive disorder occurs secondary to the diagnosis of a chronic medical condition. The stress of the medical illness itself typically induces anxiety or depression. Often, these symptoms diminish when treatment is explained and initiated, and hope is offered.

Within the context of a chronic medical condition, anxiety and depression often occur simultaneously. In general, anxiety precedes depression, and depression is more likely to persevere in individuals who also have an anxiety disorder. When anxiety and depression coexist, assessment and treatment may be more challenging, underscoring the need for an aggressive, ongoing approach to assessment and treatment.

A common but erroneous assumption by clinicians is that the psychological distress that accompanies a medical condition, even when it is severe and

---

Box 10.1 Brief Screening Measures Used in Nonpsychiatric Settings for Cognitive Functioning, Anxiety, and Depression

Folstein Mini-Mental Exam
Beck Depression Inventory
Center for Epidemiological Studies of Depression Scale
Geriatric Depression Scale
Hospital Anxiety and Depression Scale
Zung Self-Rating Depression Scale
Zung Self-Rating Anxiety Scale
PHQ9

Box 10.2 Symptoms Indicating an Anxiety Disorder in Medically Ill Patients in the Absence of Physiologic Course

Chronic apprehension, worry, inability to relax not related to illness or treatment

Difficulty concentrating

Irritability or outbursts of anger

Difficulty falling asleep or staying asleep not explained by illness or treatment

Trembling or shaking not explained by illness or treatment

Exaggerated startle response

Perspiring for no apparent reason

Chest pain or tightness in the chest

Fear of places, events, certain activities

Unrealistic fear of dying

Fear of "going crazy"

Recurrent and persistent ideas, thoughts, or impulses

Repetitive behaviors to prevent discomfort

Adapted from references 3 and 5.

---

unremitting, is natural, expected, and does not require or respond to treatment. This attitude leads to underrecognition and undertreatment of high levels of suffering. Untreated psychological symptoms can lead to post-traumatic stress disorder (PTSD).[6,8] PTSD, typically induced by exposure to extreme stress and/or trauma, is increasingly being linked in the literature to medical treatment situations. Providers are apt to confuse PTSD symptoms such as avoidance and withdrawal as nonpathologic responses (e.g., acceptance adjustment). In the treatment of PTSD, psychopharmacologic agents alone are inadequate and must be accompanied by aggressive psychotherapeutic interventions, education, and support.

Box 10.3 Symptoms Indicating a Depressive Disorder in Medically Ill Patients in the Absence of Physiologic Course

Enduring depressed or sad mood, tearful

Marked disinterest or lack of pleasure in social activities, family, and friends not explained by pain or fatigue

Feelings of worthlessness and hopelessness

Excessive enduring guilt that illness is a punishment

Significant weight loss or gain not explained by dieting, illness, or treatments

Hopelessness about the future

Enduring fatigue

Increase or decrease in sleep not explained by illness or treatment

Recurring thoughts of death or suicidal thoughts or acts

Diminished ability to think and make decisions

Adapted from references 3 and 5.

Assessment and Screening Considerations

Assessment of Anxiety

The experience of anxiety is virtually universal, especially when a person has a serious chronic illness. Anxiety is a vague, subjective feeling of apprehension, tension, insecurity, and uneasiness, usually without a known, specific cause identifiable by the individual. Box 10.2 lists anxiety symptoms that indicate a psychiatric disorder and call for psychiatric assessment and treatment. Skill in early recognition of anxiety is important so that care providers can intervene to alleviate symptoms, prevent escalation and loss of control, and enable adjustment and coping.

Assessment of Depression

Underrecognized and undertreated, depression has the potential to decrease immune response, decrease survival time, impair ability to adhere to treatment, and impair quality of life.[9] In addition to medical comorbidity, risk factors that favor the development of a depressive disorder include prior episodes of depression, family history of depression, prior suicide attempts, female gender, age under 40 years, postpartum period, lack of social support, stressful life events, personal history of sexual abuse, and current substance abuse.[5]

Cultural Considerations

Culture can be a powerful influence on the occurrence and presentation of psychiatric morbidity. In some cultures, anxiety and depression may be expressed through somatic symptoms rather than affective/behavioral symptoms such as guilt or sadness.[10] Complaints of "nerves" and headaches (in Latino and Mediterranean cultures); of weakness, tiredness, or "imbalance" (in Chinese or Asian cultures); of problems of the "heart" (in Middle Eastern cultures); or of being "heartbroken" (among the Hopi) may be depressive equivalents. Cultures may differ in judgments about the seriousness of dysphoria; for example, irritability may be a greater concern than sadness or withdrawal. Experiences distinctive to certain cultures, such as fear of being hexed or vivid feelings of being visited by those who have died, must be differentiated from actual hallucinations or delusions that may be part of a major depressive episode with psychotic features.

Screening for Anxiety and Depression

A number of tools have been developed to screen for psychological distress but have not been consistently incorporated into clinical care.

One tool that is easy to administer, reliable, and palatable to patients is the Distress Thermometer. This tool is similar to pain measurement scales that ask patients to rate their pain on a scale from 0 to 10 and consists of two cards. The first card is a picture of a thermometer, and the patient is asked to mark his or her level of distress. A rating of 5 or above indicates that a patient has symptoms indicating a need to be evaluated by a mental health professional and potential referral for services. The patient is then handed a second card and asked to identify which items from a six-item problem list relate to the patient's distress; that is, illness-related, family, emotional, practical, financial, or spiritual.

Asking "Are you depressed?" was found to be reliable and valid for diagnosing depression and is extraordinarily useful in care of the terminally ill.

Suicide

Suicide is the ninth leading cause of death in the United States. Five percent of suicides occur in patients with chronic medical illnesses, spinal cord injuries, multiple sclerosis, cancer, and HIV disease.[11]

The strongest suicide predictor is the presence of a psychiatric illness, especially depression and alcohol abuse, although a chronic deteriorating medical illness with perceived poor health, recent diagnosis of a life-threatening illness, and recent conflict or loss of a significant relationship also are considered to be predictive.[11] Being male, being older than 45 years, and living alone and lacking a social support system are risk factors. Other cancer-related risk factors include oral, pharyngeal, or lung cancer; poor prognosis; confusion and delirium; inadequately controlled pain; and the presence of deficits, such as loss of mobility, loss of bowel or bladder control, amputation, sensory loss, inability to eat or swallow, and exhaustion.[11]

The highest-risk patients are those with severe and rapidly progressive disease producing rapid functional decline, intractable pain, and/or history of depression, suicide attempts, or substance abuse.

Physician-Assisted Suicide

Whereas suicide is the intentional ending of one's own life, physician-assisted suicide (PAS) refers to a physician acting to aid a person in the ending of his or her life.[12,13] Public demand for PAS has been fueled by burdensome, exhausting, and expensive dying in acute care settings. Implications for health care providers include the following: to be knowledgeable about the legal and moral/ethical aspects of PAS; to do a personal evaluation and prepare responses for situations with patients in which the topic may arise; to improve education about pain management, symptom control, and related issues in the care of dying and seriously ill patients; to conduct rigorous research on the attitudes and practices of health care professionals with respect to assisted suicide; and to develop effective mechanisms to address conflicts.

Assessment of Suicide Risk

Assessment and treatment of depression, often overlooked in chronic illness treatment settings, is a key suicide prevention strategy. In addition, managing symptoms, communicating, and helping patients to maintain a sense of control are vitally important prevention strategies. An assessment of depression should always include the following:

- Direct questions about suicidal thinking, plans, or attempts
- Despair or hopelessness
- Distress from poorly managed symptoms
- Personal or family history of suicidal ideation, plans, or attempts[14]

When any indicator of suicide risk is recognized, there should be a thorough evaluation of risk factors, clues, suicidal ideation, level of depression, hopelessness and despair, and symptom distress in order to estimate individual lethality. Find out what method the patient is considering and whether the means are available.

Suicidal persons usually give verbal and/or behavioral clues, such as isolated or withdrawn behavior or death wishes or death themes in art, writing, play, or conversation. Clues may be subtle or obvious, for example, joking about suicide, asking questions concerning death (e.g., "How many of these pills would it take to kill someone?"), making comments with a theme of giving up, or making statements that indicate hopelessness or helplessness.

Suicide Interventions

Severely depressed and potentially suicidal patients must be identified as soon as possible to ensure a safe environment and appropriate treatment.[14] A patient with an immediate, lethal, and precise suicide plan needs strict safety precautions such as hospitalization and continuous or close supervision. Notify the primary provider and document the patient's behavior and verbatim statements, suicide assessment, and rationale for decisions, as well as the time and date the provider was notified.[14] If the provider is not responsive to the report of the patient's suicidal ideation, it is important to maintain observation and to pursue psychiatric consultation.

Management of Anxiety and Depression

Psychosocial interventions can exert an important effect on the overall adjustment of patients and their families to chronic illness and treatment. Several studies document the beneficial effect of counseling on anxiety, feelings of personal control, depression, and generalized psychological distress. Increased length of survival from time of diagnosis has highlighted the need for psychopharmacologic, psychotherapeutic, and behaviorally oriented interventions to reduce anxiety and depression and to improve quality of life for patients diagnosed with a chronic illness.

Pharmacologic Interventions

Pharmacotherapy, as an adjunct to one or more of the psychotherapies, can be an important aid in bringing psychological symptoms under control.

Pharmacologic Management of Anxiety

The following brief review of pharmacologic treatment must be supplemented with other references concerning assessment, intervention, evaluation, and patient education (Box 10.4).[3]

Benzodiazepines are the most frequently used medication for anxiety in both medical and psychiatric settings. When longer-acting benzodiazepines, such as diazepam, are used in elderly patients or in the presence of liver disease, dosages should be decreased and dosing intervals increased. They may suppress respiratory drive. Consultation-liaison services often use lorazepam in medically ill patients because its elimination half-life is relatively unaffected by liver disease, age, or concurrent use of selective serotonin reuptake inhibitors (SSRIs) or nefazodone. Drawbacks include amnestic episodes and

> **Box 10.4 Selected Medications Commonly Used for the Treatment of Anxiety in Medically Ill Patients**
>
> **Benzodiazepines**
>
> Diazepam (Valium and others)
> Alprazolam (Xanax)
> Clonazepam (Klonopin)
> Lorazepam (Ativan and others)
> Oxazepam (Serax and others)
>
> **Azapirones**
>
> Buspirone (Buspar)
>
> **Cyclic Antidepressants**
>
> Nortriptyline (Pamelor and others)
>
> **Other Antidepressants**
>
> Fluoxetine (Prozac), a selective serotonin reuptake inhibitor (SSRI)
> Sertraline (Zoloft), an SSRI
> Paroxetine (Paxil), an SSRI
> Citalopram (Celexa) an SSRI
> Escitalopram (Lexapro) an SSRI
> Duloxetine (Cymbalta) an SNRI
> Venlafaxine (Effexor), an SNRI
> Mirtazapine (Remeron)
>
> **Other Medications Selectively Used for Their Anxiolytic Effects**
>
> β-Adrenergic blocking agents, such as propranolol
> Neuroleptics (antipsychotics), such as olanzapine (Zyprexa), Quetiapine (Seroquel)

interdose anxiety caused by its short half-life. The latter can be remedied by more frequent dosing. If medically ill patients need a longer-acting benzodiazepine for panic disorder or generalized anxiety disorder, clonazepam is often used because it is not affected by concurrent use of SSRIs. Clonazepam may accumulate and result in oversedation and ataxia in elderly patients; therefore, low doses are used. Temazepam is useful as a sedative-hypnotic.

Buspirone, used primarily for generalized anxiety disorder, is preferable for anxiety in medically ill patients because of its lack of sedation, lack of negative effects on cognition, insignificant effect of age on elimination half-life, and limited effect of liver disease on half-life. Buspirone has almost no clinically significant interactions with drugs commonly used in general medicine. It may stimulate the respiratory drive, which makes it useful in patients with pulmonary disease or sleep apnea.

Cyclic antidepressants are well established as anxiolytic agents, which are particularly effective in the treatment of panic disorder and in generalized anxiety disorder. Potentially deleterious side effects in medically ill patients are sedative, anticholinergic, orthostatic hypotensive, and quinidine-like. Liver disease and renal disease may affect metabolism and excretion of the drug, and therefore, it requires careful dosage titration.

Other drugs that may be used for anxiety include the β-adrenergic blocking agents, antihistamines, monoamine oxidase inhibitors, and neuroleptics. β-Adrenergic blocking agents may be used for milder forms of generalized anxiety, but there are cautions and contraindications in the presence of pulmonary disease, diabetes, and congestive heart failure. Antihistamines are sometimes used, although the effects are largely nonspecific and sedative. Side effects, such as sedation and dizziness, can be significant for medically ill patients. Monoamine oxidase inhibitors are rarely used in medically ill patients because of the precautions that must be taken to prevent drug interactions.

Neuroleptics, such as haloperidol in low doses, are used for anxiety associated with severe behavioral agitation or psychotic symptoms.

Pharmacologic Management of Depression

Medical illnesses and the medications required to treat or manage symptoms may impose significantly modified prescribing regimens on the use of antidepressants (Box 10.5).[15] Therefore, it is necessary to evaluate the possible role

---

Box 10.5 Selected Medications Used for the Treatment of Depression in Medically Ill Patients

Selective Serotonin Reuptake Inhibitors

Sertraline (Zoloft)
Paroxetine (Paxil)
Citalopram (Celexa)
Escitalopram (Lexapro)

Serotonin/Norepinephrine Reuptake Inhibitors

Venlafaxine (Effexor)
Duloxetine (Cymbalta)

Tricyclic Antidepressants

Desipramine (Norpramin)
Nortriptyline (Aventyl, Pamelor)

Noradrenergic Agonist

Mirtazapine (Remeron)

Psychostimulants

Methylphenidate
Provigil (Modafinil)

Dopamine Reuptake Blocking Compounds

Bupropion (Wellbutrin, Zyban)

Adapted from Beliles K, Stoudemire A. Psychopharmacologic treatment of depression in the medically ill. *Psychosomatics.* 1998;39:S2–S19.

of existing medical conditions and medications that could cause the depressive symptoms.

Other general guidelines include the following:

1. Use the medication with the least potential for drug–drug interactions and for adverse effects based on the patient's drug regimen and physiologic vulnerabilities, and with the greatest potential for improving the primary symptoms of the depression.

2. Begin with low dosage, increase slowly, and establish the lowest effective dosage.

3. Reassess dosage requirements regularly.

The SSRIs have fewer long-term side effects than the tricyclic antidepressants and, in general, are the first line of pharmacologic antidepressant treatment unless specific side-effect profiles associated with other classes of drugs are desired.

Psychostimulants, such as methylphenidate, have been useful in the treatment of depression in medically ill patients. Advantages include rapid onset of action and rapid clearance if side effects occur. They can also counteract opioid-induced sedation and improve pain control through a positive action on mood.

Antidepressant medications may take 2 to 6 weeks to produce their desired effects. Patients may need ongoing support, reassurance, and monitoring before experiencing the antidepressant effects of medication. Patient education is essential in this area to decrease the possibility of nonadherence to the medication regimen.

Psychotherapeutic Modalities

Psychosocial interventions are defined as systematic efforts applied to influence coping behavior through educational or psychotherapeutic means. The goals of such interventions are to improve morale, self-esteem, coping ability, sense of control, and problem-solving abilities and to decrease emotional distress. The educational approach is directive, using problem-solving and cognitive methods. Psychotherapeutic interventions, as opposed to educational interventions, should be delivered by professionals with special training in both mental health and specific interventional modalities as applied to patients with chronic medical illnesses and palliative care needs.

Psychotherapeutic Interventions Targeted to Symptoms of Anxiety

Anxiety responses can be thought of as occurring along a continuum, from mild to moderate to severe to panic. As a person moves along the continuum to moderate, severe, and panic levels of anxiety, the problem-causing distress is lost sight of, and distress itself becomes the focus of attention. Both preventive and treatment strategies can be used with patients and family members in a variety of settings.

- Asking whether the patient was taking medications for "nerves," depression, or insomnia will help to determine whether drugs were inappropriately discontinued, or whether anxiety symptoms predated the current illness.

- In addition, ask about over-the-counter medications, illegal drugs, alcohol intake, and smoking history. Documentation and communication of findings are essential to enhance teamwork among providers.
- Frequently, patients can identify the factors causing their anxiety, as well as coping skills effective in the past, and when they do, their discomfort decreases.
- Use open-ended questions, reflection, clarification, and/or empathic remarks, such as "You're afraid of being a burden?" to help the patient to identify previously effective coping strategies and to integrate them with new ones.
- Use statements such as, "What has helped you get through difficult times like this before?" "How can we help you use those strategies now?" or "How about talking about some new strategies that may work now?"

Preventive and Treatment Strategies to Address Anxiety

Preventive strategies can help to maintain a useful level of anxiety, one that enhances rather than interferes with problem solving (Table 10.3).

Table 10.3 Hierarchy of Anxiety Interventions

Anxiety Level	Interventions
Level 1	*Prevention strategies*
Mild to moderate	Provide concrete objective information.
	Ensure stressful-event warning.
	Increase opportunities for control.
	Increase patient and family participation in care activities.
	Acknowledge fears.
	Explore near-miss events, past and/or present.
	Control symptoms.
	Structure uncertainty.
	Limit sensory deprivation and isolation.
	Encourage hope.
Level 2	*Treatment strategies*
Moderate to severe	Use presence of support person as "emotional anchor."
	Support expression of feelings, doubts, and fears.
	Explore near-miss events, past and/or present.
	Provide accurate information for realistic restructuring of fearful ideas.
	Teach anxiety-reduction strategies, such as focusing, breathing, relaxation, and imagery techniques.

(continued)

Table 10.3 (Continued)

Anxiety Level	Interventions
	Use massage, touch, and physical exercise. Control symptoms. Use antianxiety medications. Delay procedures to promote patient control and readiness. Consult psychiatric experts.
Level 3	*Treatment strategies*
Panic	Stay with the patient. Maintain calm environment and reduce stimulation. Use antianxiety medications and monitor carefully. Control symptoms. Use focusing and breathing techniques. Use demonstration in addition to verbal direction. Repeat realistic reassurances. Communicate with repetition and simplicity. Consult psychiatric experts.

Adapted from Minarik P. Psychosocial intervention with ineffective coping responses to physical illness: depression-related. In: Barry PD, ed. *Psychosocial Nursing: Care of Physically Ill Patients and Their Families.* New York: Lippincott-Raven, 1996:323–339.

Table 10.4 Nonpharmacologic Interventions for Treatment of Depression

Cognitive Interventions	Behavioral Interventions
Review and reinforce realistic ideas and expectations.	Provide directed activities.
Help the patient test the accuracy of self-defeating assumptions.	Develop a hierarchy of behaviors with the patient and use a graded task assignment.
Help the patient identify and test negative automatic thoughts.	
Review and reinforce the patient's strengths.	Develop structured daily activity schedules.
Set realistic, achievable goals.	Encourage the at-home use of a diary or journal to monitor automatic thoughts, behaviors, and emotions; review this with the patient.
Explain all actions and plans, seek feedback and participation in decision making.	
Provide choices (e.g., about the timing of an activity).	Use systematic application of reinforcement.

(continued)

Table 10.4 (Continued)

Cognitive Interventions	Behavioral Interventions
Teach thought stopping or thought interruption to halt negative or self-defeating thoughts.	Encourage self-monitoring of predetermined behaviors, such as sleep pattern, diet, and physical exercises.
Encourage exploration of feelings only for a specific purpose and only if the patient is not ruminating (e.g., constant repeating of failures or problems).	Focus on goal attainment and preparation for future adaptive coping.
Direct the patient to activities with gentle reminders to focus as a way to discourage rumination.	**Specific behavioral strategies**
	Observe the patient's self-care patterns, then negotiate with the patient to develop a structured, daily schedule.
Listen and take appropriate action on physical complaints, then redirect and assist the patient to accomplish activities.	Develop realistic daily self-care goals with the patient to increase sense of control.
Avoid denying the patient's sadness or depressed feelings or reason to feel that way.	Upgrade the goals gradually to provide increased opportunity for positive reinforcement and goal attainment.
Avoid chastising the patient for feeling sad.	
	Use a chart for monitoring daily progress; gold stars may be used as reinforcement; a visible chart facilitates communication, consistency among caregivers, and meaningful reinforcement (i.e., praise and positive attention from others).
Interpersonal interventions	
Educate the patient about the physical and biochemical causes of depression and the good prognosis.	
Enhance social skills through modeling, role-playing, rehearsal, feedback, and reinforcement.	Provide sufficient time and repetitive reassurance ("You can do it") to encourage patients to accomplish self-care actions.
Build rapport with frequent, short visits.	
Engage in normal social conversation with the patient as often as possible.	Positively reinforce even small achievements.
Give consistent attention, even when the patient is uncommunicative, to show that the patient is worthwhile.	Provide physical assistance with self-care activities, especially those related to appearance and hygiene, that the patient is unable to do.
Direct comments and questions to the patient rather than to significant others.	
Allow adequate time for the patient to prepare a response.	Adjust physical assistance, verbal direction, reminders, and teaching to the actual needs and abilities of the patient; avoid increasing unnecessary dependence by overdoing.

(continued)

Table 10.4 (Continued)

Cognitive Interventions	Behavioral Interventions
Mobilize family and social support systems.	
Encourage the patient to maintain open communication and share feelings with significant others.	Teach deep-breathing or relaxation techniques for anxiety management.
Supportively involve family and friends and teach them how to help.	
Avoid sharing with the patient your personal reactions to the patient's dependent behavior.	**Complementary therapies**
	Guided imagery and visualization
Avoid medical jargon, advice giving, sharing personal experiences, or making value judgments.	Art and music therapies
	Humor
Avoid false reassurance.	Aerobic exercise
	Phototherapy
	Aromatherapy and massage

Adapted from Minarik P. Psychosocial intervention with ineffective coping responses to physical illness: depression-related. In: Barry PD, ed. *Psychosocial Nursing: Care of Physically Ill Patients and Their Families.* New York: Lippincott-Raven, 1996:323–339.

Psychotherapeutic Interventions Targeted to Symptoms of Depression

Depression is inadequately treated in palliative care, although many patients experience depressive symptoms. Goals for the depressed patient are as follows:

1. To ensure a safe environment
2. To assist the patient in reducing depressive symptoms and maladaptive coping responses
3. To restore or increase the patient's functional level
4. To improve quality of life, if possible
5. To prevent future relapse and recurrence of depression

Table 10.4 lists nonpharmacologic interventions designed to address a variety of techniques used to treat depression.[16]

Conclusion

The psychosocial issues in persons facing life-threatening illness are influenced by individual, sociocultural, medical, and family factors. Most patients receiving palliative treatment, and their families, experience expected periods of emotional turmoil that occur at transition points, as is seen, for example, along the clinical course of cancer. Some patients experience anxiety and depressive disorders. Assessment and treatment of psychosocial problems, including physical symptoms, psychological distress, caregiver burden, and psychiatric disorders, can enhance quality of life throughout the palliative care trajectory.

References

1. Kirkova J, Walsh D, Rybicki L, et al. Symptom severity and distress in advanced cancer. *Palliat Med.* 2010;24:330–339.

2. Hsu T, Ennis M, Hood N, et al. Quality of life in long-term breast cancer survivors. *J Clin Oncol.* 2013;31(28):3540–3548.

3. Holland JC, Alici Y. Management of distress in cancer patients. *J Support Oncol.* 2010;8(1):4–12.

4. van Laarhoven HW, Schilderman J, Bleijenberg G, et al. Coping, quality of life, depression, and hopelessness in cancer patients in a curative and palliative, end-of-life care setting. *Cancer Nurs.* 2011;34(4):302–314.

5. Walker J, Holm Hansen C, Martin P, et al. Prevalence of depression in adults with cancer: a systematic review. *Ann Oncol.* 2013;24(4):895–900.

6. Seitz DC, Besier T, Debatin KM, et al. Posttraumatic stress, depression and anxiety among adult long-term survivors of cancer in adolescence. *Eur J Cancer.* 2010;46(9):1596–1606.

7. Fitch MI. Screening for distress: a role for oncology nursing. *Curr Opin Oncol.* 2011;23(4):331–337.

8. Rustad JK, David D, Currier MB. Cancer and post-traumatic stress disorder: diagnosis, pathogenesis, and treatment considerations. *Palliat Support Care.* 2012;10:213–223.

9. Lutgendorf SK, Sood AK. Biobehavioral factors and cancer progression: physiological pathways and mechanisms. *Psychosom Med.* 2011;73(9):724–730.

10. Wright AA, Stieglitz H, Kupersztoch YM, et al. United States acculturation and cancer patients' end-of-life care. *PLoS One.* 2013;8(3):e58663.

11. Misono S, Weiss NS, Fann JR, et al. Incidence of suicide in persons with cancer. *J Clin Oncol.* 2008;26(29):4731–4738.

12. Hendry M, Pasterfield D, Lewis R, et al. Whyd do we want the right to die? A systematic review of the international literature on the views of patients, carers and the public on assisted dying. *Palliat Med.* 2013;27(1):13–26.

13. Steck N, Egger M, Maessen M, et al. Euthanasia and assisted suicide in selected European countries and US states: systematic literature review. *Med Care.* 2013;51(10):938–944.

14. Cooke L, Gotto J, Mayorga L, et al. What do I say? Suicide assessment and management. *Clin J Oncol Nurs.* 2013;17(1):E1–7.

15. Beliles K, Stoudemire A. Psychopharmacologic treatment of depression in the medically ill. *Psychosomatics.* 1998;39:S2–S19.

16. Minarik P. Psychosocial intervention with ineffective coping responses to physical illness: depression-related. In: Barry PD, ed. *Psychosocial Nursing: Care of Physically Ill Patients and Their Families.* New York: Lippincott-Raven, 1996:323–339.

Chapter 11

Insomnia

Laura Bourdeanu, Marjorie J. Hein, and Ellen A. Liu

Introduction

Insomnia is a prevalent health complaint, with an estimated 6% to 10% of Americans suffering from insomnia on a regular basis each year.[1] Insomnia is predominant among elderly people, people with chronic medical illness, and those with anxiety or depressive disorders. Unchecked, insomnia can lead to various adverse sequelae in psychiatric, neurocognitive, and medical domains, as well as significant reduction in quality of life. In addition, insomnia can lead to daytime dysfunction, such as daytime sleepiness, irritability, depressive or anxious mood, and accidents.

In patients with cancer, insomnia is reported to be a common problem. The causes for insomnia in patients with cancer may be related to psychological factors (anxiety or depression), pain, treatment-related toxicity, or other comorbid medical conditions. Further, insomnia is linked with increased rates of depression, decreased quality of life, and increased fatigue in other patient populations.[2] Consequences of insomnia are listed in Box 11.1.

Factors Related to Insomnia

Insomnia is among one of the most prevalent, distressing, and undermanaged symptoms. Insomnia is associated with adverse outcomes and should be proactively targeted for intervention. Often, sleep disturbances are associated with situational stresses such as illness, aging, and drug treatments.[2] However, the physical illness, pain, hospitalization, and medications, along with the psychological impact of a life-threatening disease, may disrupt sleeping patterns. A history of poor sleep patterns will adversely affect the individual's daytime mood and performance. Among the general population, an individual with complaints of persistent insomnia has been associated with an increased risk for developing anxiety or depression. Complaints of sleep disturbances and a pattern of sleep-wake cycle reversals may be an early sign of a developing delirium.[3]

Paraneoplastic syndromes may exacerbate sleep disturbances if they are associated with increased steroid production and if the patient has symptoms associated with tumor invasion such as draining lesions, gastrointestinal and genitourinary changes, pain, fever, cough, dyspnea, pruritus, and fatigue.

Box 11.1 Potential Consequences of Insomnia in the Context of Cancer

Psychological and Behavioral Consequences

Fatigue

Cognitive impairments (e.g., memory, concentration)

Mood disturbances and psychiatric disorders

Psychological and Health Consequences

Health problems and physical symptoms (e.g., pain)

Longevity

Immunosuppression

Adapted from Savard J, Villa J, Ivers H, et al. Prevalence, natural course, and risk factors of insomnia comorbid with cancer over a 2-month period. *J Clin Oncol*. 2009;27(31):5233–5239.

Moreover, medications used by patients to control symptoms of the disease or side effects of treatment may cause insomnia. For example, medications such as vitamins, corticosteroids, neuroleptics for nausea and vomiting, and sympathomimetics to relieve dyspnea may negatively affect sleep patterns. Frequently, hospitalized patients are likely to have their sleep interrupted by treatment schedules, routine hospital procedures, and other patients sharing the room. All of these factors may either singularly or collectively alter the sleep-wake cycle. Other considerations influencing the sleep-wake cycles of patients with cancer include age, comfort, pain, anxiety, environmental noise, and temperature.

There are four major categories of sleep disorders according to the Sleep Disorders Classification Committee of the American Academy of Sleep Medicine:

1. Disorders of initiating and maintaining sleep (insomnias)

2. Disorders of the sleep-wake cycle

3. Dysfunctions associated with sleep, sleep stages, or partial arousals (parasomnias)

4. Disorders of excessive somnolence[4]

According to the *Diagnostic and Statistical Manual of Mental Disorders*, fourth edition text revision (DSM-IV-TR), sleep disorders are organized into four major categories according to the etiology of the sleep disorder[5]:

1. Primary sleep disorders are those with etiologies other than the ones listed in categories 2 to 4 above. Primary sleep disorders are assumed to develop from endogenous abnormalities in sleep-wake patterns, accompanied by conditioning factors.

   a. Dyssomnias are abnormalities in the amount, quality, or timing of sleep.

   b. Parasomnias are abnormal behavioral or physiologic events.

2. Sleep disorder related to another mental disorder resulting from a diagnosable mental disorder, usually mood or anxiety disorder, but severe enough to receive clinical attention

3. Sleep disorder due to a general medical condition resulting from the effects of a physiologic medical condition
4. Substance-induced sleep disorder resulting from concurrent use or a recent discontinuation of a drug

Insomnia may also be caused by medications:

- Central nervous system (CNS) stimulants such as amphetamines, psychostimulants used to treat attention deficit disorders (e.g., methylphenidate), caffeine, and diet pills (including some dietary supplements that promote weight loss and appetite suppression)
- Sedatives and hypnotics (e.g., glutethimide, benzodiazepines, pentobarbital, chloral hydrate, secobarbital sodium, and amobarbital sodium)
- Cancer chemotherapeutic agents (especially antimetabolites)
- Anticonvulsants (e.g., phenytoin)
- Adrenocorticotropin
- Oral contraceptives
- Monoamine oxidase inhibitors
- Methyldopa
- Propranolol
- Atenolol
- Alcohol
- Thyroid preparations

In addition, withdrawal from CNS depressants (e.g., barbiturates, opioids, glutethimide, chloral hydrate, methaqualone, alcohol, and over-the-counter and prescription antihistamine sedatives), benzodiazepines, major tranquilizers, tricyclic and monoamine oxidase inhibitor antidepressants, and illicit drugs (e.g., marijuana, cocaine, phencyclidine) can cause insomnia.

Perpetuating Factors

Cognitive and behavioral mechanisms perpetuate insomnia, regardless of how insomnia is triggered. Patients have misconceptions about what are normal sleep requirements and then develop excessive worry about not having adequate sleep. This often causes the patient to become obsessive about sleep. The patient develops a dysfunctional belief, often worsening the disruptive sleep behavior—for example, taking daytime naps or "sleeping in late"—which in turn reduces the natural homeostatic drive to sleep at a normal bedtime.

Patients develop a conditioned arousal to stimuli that would normally be associated with sleep (i.e., heightened anxiety and ruminations about going to sleep once they are in the bedroom). Patients then develops a cycle in which the more they strive to sleep, the more agitated they become, and the less they are able to fall asleep. Also, the patient may have ruminative thoughts or clock-watching behavior as they try to fall asleep in the bedroom. Therefore, conditioned environmental stimuli cause insomnia to develop from the continued association of sleeplessness with situations and behaviors that are typically related to sleep.

In addition, prescription drug use, somatic disorders, neurologic declined, reduced exposure to outdoor light, polyphasic sleep-wake patterns, and lack of physical activity perpetuate the greater prevalence of insomnia in elderly individuals.

Treatment

Insomnia may be due to a variety of disease-related factors, cancer treatment, or psychological factors. The initial strategy to treat insomnia in cancer patients is to address the underlying physical and psychological factors contributing to the sleep disturbance. If the precipitating factors are not fully manageable, then pharmacologic or behavioral interventions, or both, should be used to treat both acute and chronic insomnia. Pharmacologic interventions are more commonly used; however, long-term pharmacotherapy is not desirable.[6] Hence, the treatment for insomnia must be multimodal and should include both pharmacologic and nonpharmacologic interventions.

Pharmacologic Interventions

Pharmacological agents approved by the U.S. Food and Drug Administration (FDA) for the treatment of insomnia include benzodiazepine γ-aminobutyric acid ($GABA_A$) agonists, nonbenzodiazepine $GABA_A$ agonists, melatonin receptor agonists, and histamine receptor antagonists (Table 11.1).[1,6]

Benzodiazepine Receptor Agonists

Benzodiazepines are still frequently used in the management of insomnia because of their undisputed efficacy and relative safety compared with other agents such as barbiturates. Although benzodiazepines are effective agents, they have several unwanted side effects, such as daytime drowsiness, dizziness or light-headedness, cognitive impairments, motor incoordination, tolerance, dependence, rebound insomnia, and daytime anxiety.[6]

Nonbenzodiazepine Receptor Agonists

Nonbenzodiazepines are the most widely used medications because they can induce sleep with fewer side effects than benzodiazepines. Although both nonbenzodiazepines and benzodiazepines exert their effect on the GABA receptor complex, nonbenzodiazepines do not disturb the architecture of sleep. Nonbenzodiazepines have fewer residual side effects, including a lower risk for abuse and dependence, less psychomotor impairment, amnesia, and daytime somnolence.[6]

Melatonin Receptor Agonists

Melatonin receptor agonists have the advantage of having minimal side effects and no potential for abuse or dependence.[6]

Histamine Receptor Antagonists

Histamine receptor antagonists, such as doxepin, are tricyclic antidepressants that are used for improving sleep-maintenance insomnia. Doxepin, the only FDA-approved drug in this class, has affinity for the H_1 histaminic receptor, which produces sedating effects. Doxepin does not produce residual effects

Table 11.1 Pharmacologic Agents Used to Treat Insomnia

Drug	Name	Dose	Contraindications
Benzodiazepine receptor agonists	Clonazepam	≥0.5 mg	Hypersensitivity, liver disease, acute open-angle glaucoma
	Lorazepam	≥0.5mg	Hypersensitivity, acute narrow-angle glaucoma, sleep apnea syndrome, severe respiratory insufficiency, given intraarterially
	Oxazepam	≥10mg	Hypersensitivity, psychoses
	Estazolam	≥1mg	Pregnancy, with ketoconazole and itraconazole
	Flurazepam	≥15mg	Hypersensitivity
	Temazepam	≥7.5mg	Pregnancy
	Triazolam	≥0.125mg	Hypersensitivity, pregnancy with ketoconazole, itraconazole, and nefazodone, medications that significantly impair the oxidative metabolism mediated by cytochrome P450 3A (CYP 3A)
	Quazepam	≥7.5mg	Hypersensitivity, sleep apnea, or with pulmonary insufficiency
Nonbenzodiazepine receptor agonists	Zaleplon	≥5mg	Hypersensitivity
	Zolpidem	≥5mg	Hypersensitivity
Melatonin receptor agonists	Zolpidem (extended release)	≥6.25mg	Hypersensitivity
Histamine receptor antagonists	Eszopiclone	≥2mg	Hypersensitivity
	Ramelton	≥8mg	Hypersensitivity, with fluvoxamine
	Doxepin	≥6mg	Hypersensitivity, glaucoma, or a tendency for urinary retention

in part because of rising levels of histamines in the morning, which override the sedative effects of doxepin in the morning. Doxepin in low doses (≤6 mg) has been shown to improve wake after sleep onset, total sleep time, and sleep efficiency.

Others

Other classes of drugs have been used to treat insomnia in cancer patients, including antidepressants, antihistamines, atypical antipsychotic agents, and neuroleptics.

- Antidepressants are increasingly used for the management of insomnia. Specifically, tricyclic antidepressants, such as amitriptyline or doxepin, trazodone, and mirtazapine, may provide sedation in patients who are not depressed, as well as those who are depressed.

- Antihistamines such as diphenhydramine and hydroxyzine are used for their sedative properties as well as for their anticholinergic properties to treat insomnia and help relieve nausea and vomiting.
- Atypical antipsychotics, such as clozapine, have been used for their sedating effects and their ability to improve appetite and relieve opioid-induced nausea.
- Neuroleptics, such as thioridazine, have been found to promote sleep, especially in patients with insomnia associated with organic mental syndrome and delirium.[2]

Nonpharmacologic Interventions

Several nonpharmacologic interventions have been used for the treatment of insomnia in healthy patients, but more intervention studies are needed to address insomnia in patients with cancer. Currently, there are four categories of nonpharmacologic interventions for insomnia: cognitive-behavioral therapies, complementary therapies, psychoeducation and information, and exercise.

Cognitive-Behavioral Therapies
Cognitive-behavioral therapies involve a variety of behavioral and psychological treatments aimed at changing negative thought processes, attitudes, and behaviors related to a person's ability to fall asleep, stay asleep, get enough sleep, and function during the day. Cognitive-behavioral therapies include the following:

- Stimulus control
- Sleep restriction
- Relaxation therapy
- Sleep hygiene
- Profile-tailored cognitive-behavioral therapy
- Cognitive restructuring strategies

These therapies have been shown to produce significantly higher quality, longer duration, and higher efficiency sleep.

Complementary Therapies
Complementary therapies are interventions that are not considered to be part of conventional medicine. Several complementary therapies have been tested:

- Aromatherapy
- Expressive therapy
- Expressive writing
- Healing
- Autogenic training
- Massage
- Muscle relaxation
- Mindfulness–based stress reduction
- Yoga

These therapies have resulted in improvement in sleep quality, duration, and efficiency; use of fewer medications; and less daytime dysfunction.[7]

Herbal Therapies

Several herbal supplements are being used for managing insomnia, especially chamomile, hops, lavender, passion flower, wild lettuce, California poppy, kava kava, St. John's wort, lemon balm, and melatonin. However they have not undergone rigorous clinical trials to determine efficacy and side effects of taking these compounds.

Psychoeducation

Psychoeducation includes the use of structured education provided to patients with specific information regarding treatments and side effects.

Exercise Interventions

Exercise interventions involve any planned, structured, and repetitive bodily movement that is performed for the purpose of conditioning any part of the body, improving health, or maintaining fitness. Several studies evaluated the efficacy of exercise intervention for the treatment of insomnia in patients with cancer, and patients reported less difficulty sleeping and improved sleep patterns and quality.[8]

Conclusion

Insomnia remains a common and distressing complaint in patients with cancer, in cancer survivors, and in those with chronic debilitating diseases. Insomnia has been linked to psychological and/or physiologic malfunction. The importance of healthy sleep in patients who are chronically ill cannot be overestimated. Effective management of insomnia begins with a thorough assessment that will include the exploration of predisposing factors such as insomnia before diagnosis, usual sleep patterns, emotional status, exercise and activity level, and other disease-related symptoms and medications. Typically, insomnia is treated with hypnotic drugs; however, more recent findings support the use of cognitive-behavioral therapies, complementary therapies, psychoeducation and information, and exercise to treat insomnia. Palliative care nurses must provide patients with education regarding healthy sleep patterns.

References

1. Morin, CM, Benca R. Chronic insomnia. *Lancet.* 2012;*379*(9821):1129–1141.

2. Savard J, Villa J, Ivers H, et al. Prevalence, natural course, and risk factors of insomnia comorbid with cancer over a 2-month period. *J Clin Oncol.* 2009;*27*(31):5233–5239.

3. Cerejeira J, Mukaetova-Ladinska E. A clinical update on delirium: from early recognition to effective management. *Nurs Res Pract.* 2011;*2011*:875176.

4. Schutte-Rodin S, Broch L, Buysse D, et al. Clinical guideline for the evaluation and management of chronic insomnia in adults. *J Clin Sleep Med.* 2008;*4*(5):487–504.

5. American Psychiatric Association. *Diagnostic and Statistical Manual of Mental Disorders,* 4th ed. Washington, DC: American Psychiatric Association, 2000.

6. Roehrs T, Roth T. Insomnia pharmacotherapy. *Neurotherapeutics.* 2012;9:728–738.

7. Sarris J, Byrne GJ. A systematic review of insomnia and complementary medicine. *Sleep Med Rev.* 2011;*15*(2):99–106.

8. Tang M, Liou T, Lin C. Improving sleep quality for cancer patients: benefits of a home-based exercise intervention. *Support Care Cancer.* 2010;*18*(10):132 9–1339.

Index